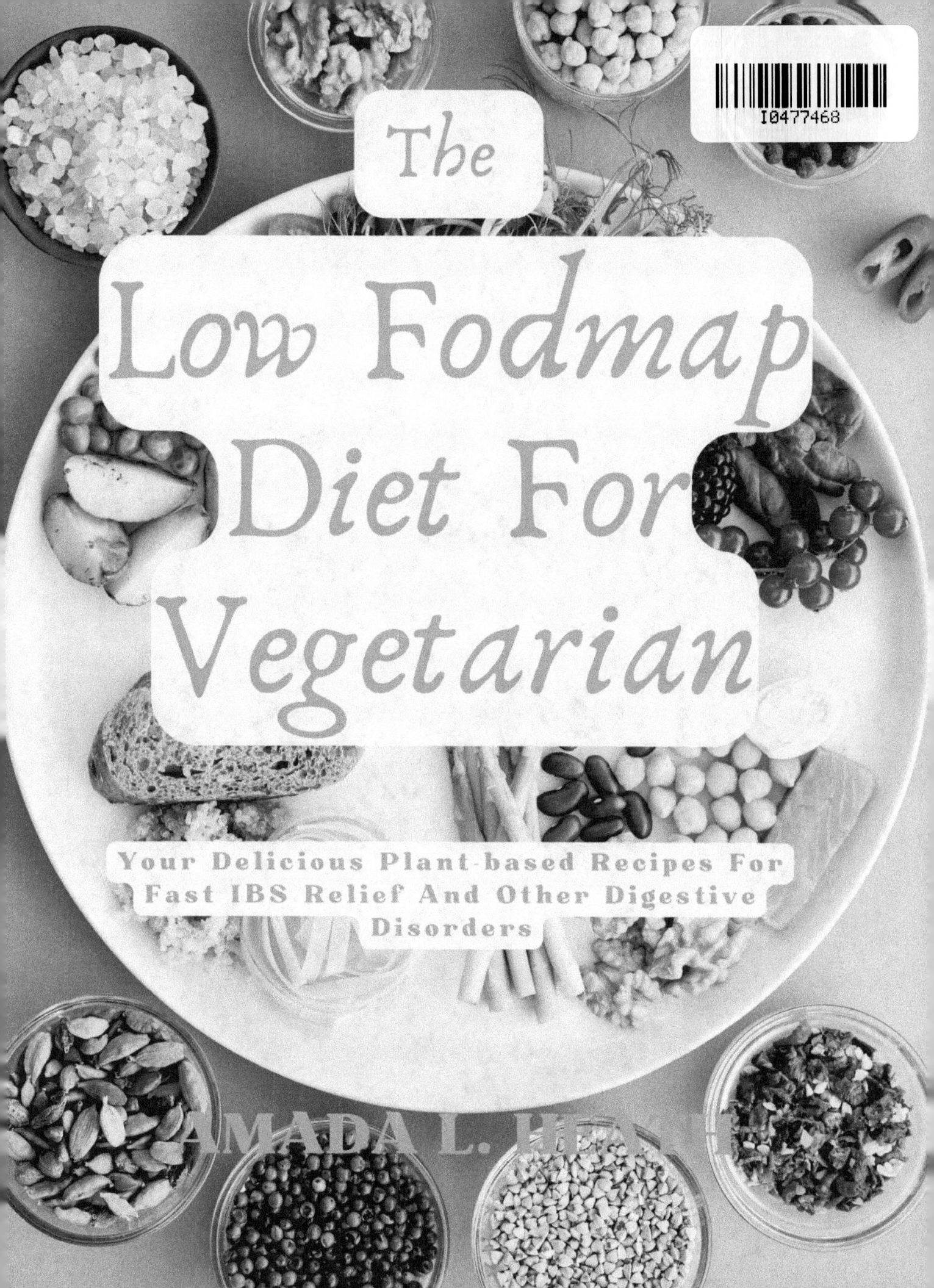

The
Low Fodmap
Diet For
Vegetarian

Your Delicious Plant-based Recipes For Fast IBS Relief And Other Digestive Disorders

AMADA L. HEART

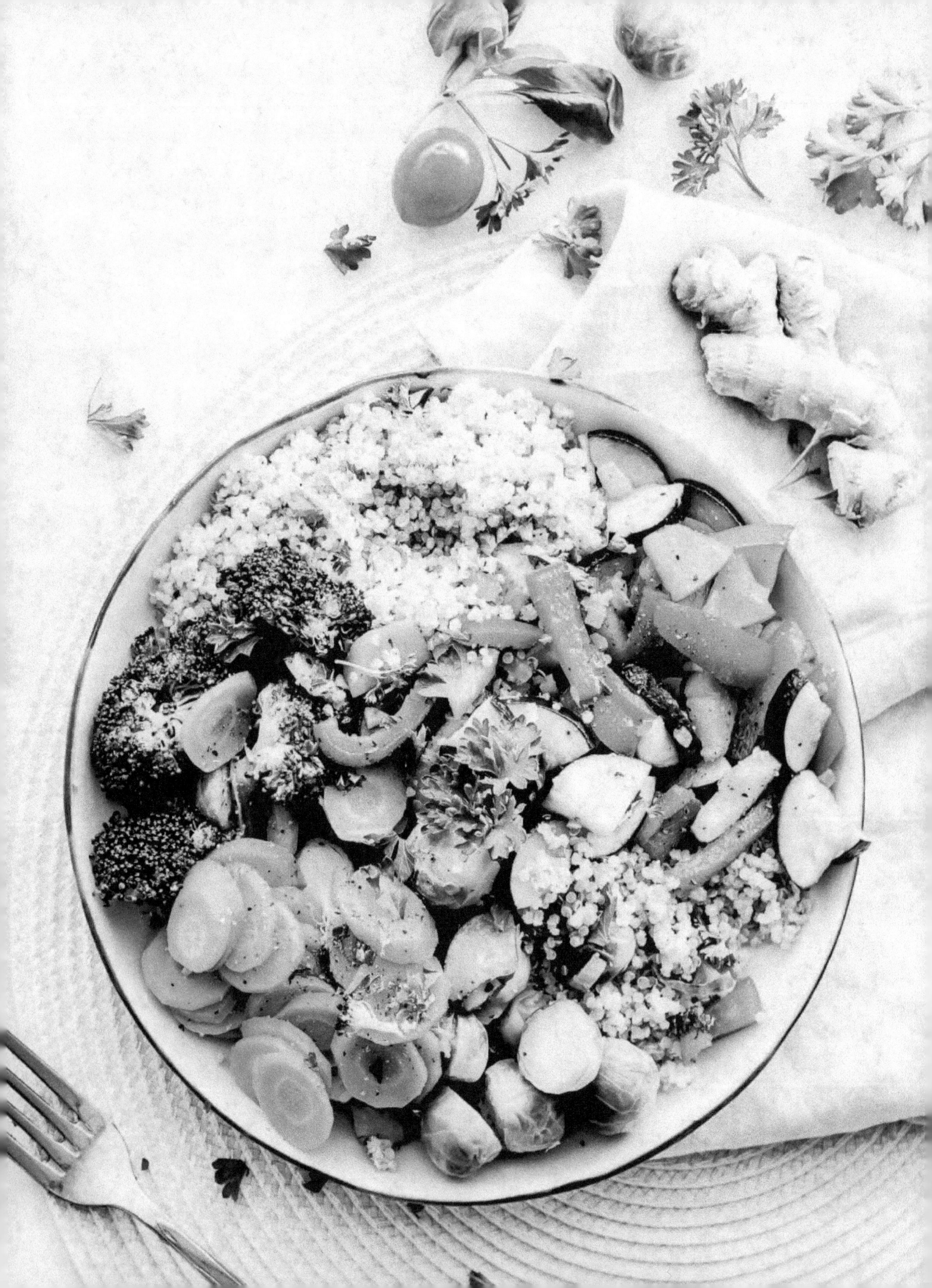

copyright

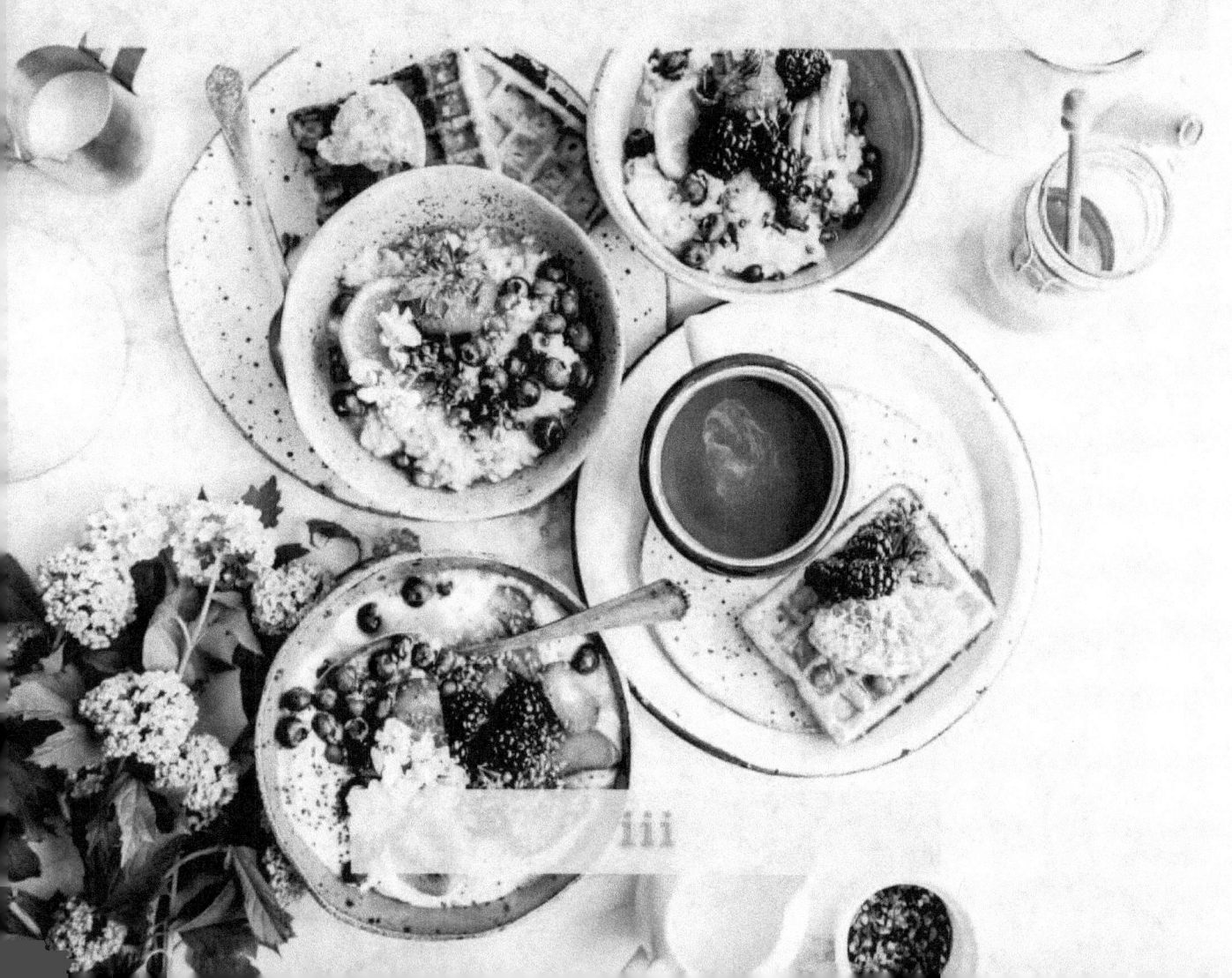

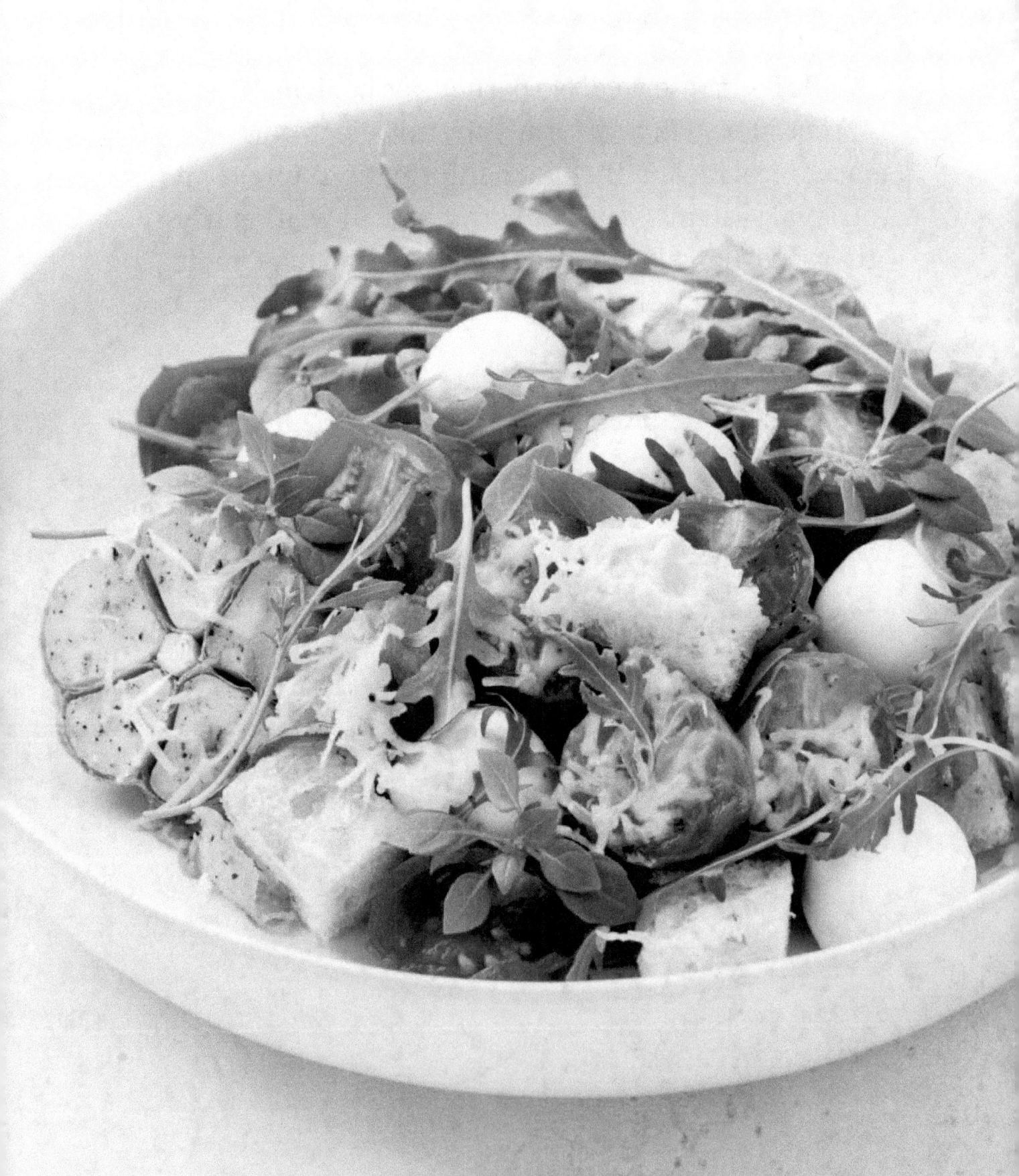

Table Of Contents

Healthy Friendly Recipes

BREAKFAST

- Banana Oat Pancakes
- Tofu Scramble
- Chia Pudding
- Quinoa Porridge
- Smoothie Bowl
- Zucchini Fritters
- Coconut Yogurt with Berries
- Pumpkin Oatmeal
- Avocado Toast
- Buckwheat Pancakes
- Polenta Porridge
- Sweet Potato Breakfast Hash
- Eggplant Breakfast Wrap
- Peanut Butter Chia Toast
- Berry Coconut Smoothie
- Buckwheat Porridge
- Overnight Oats
- Gluten-Free Waffles
- Coconut Rice Porridge
- Low-FODMAP Granola

LUNCH

- Grilled Vegetable Quinoa Salad
- Vegetarian Stuffed Bell Peppers
- Zucchini Noodles with Pesto
- Tofu Stir-Fry with Bok Choy
- Cucumber Avocado Salad
- Lentil and Spinach Soup
- Vegetable Stir-Fry with Rice
- Grilled Eggplant with Chickpeas
- Avocado Chickpea Wrap
- Roasted Vegetable Tacos
- Quinoa and Roasted Veggie Bowl
- Spinach and Feta Stuffed Portobello Mushrooms
- Rice Noodle Stir-Fry
- Stuffed Zucchini Boats
- Eggplant and Lentil Stew
- Sweet Potato and Chickpea Salad
- Grilled Tofu with Veggies
- Vegetarian Taco Salad
- Tomato and Avocado Wrap
- Coconut Curry Vegetables

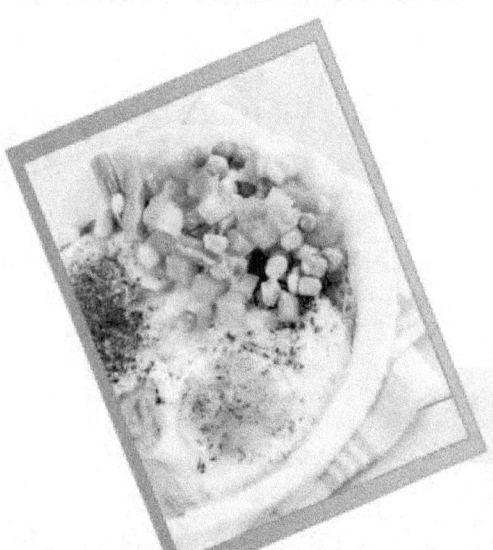

DINNER

- Vegetarian Stir-Fry with Tofu
- Vegetable Lentil Curry
- Stuffed Bell Peppers with Quinoa
- Eggplant Stir-Fry
- Zucchini and Mushroom Risotto
- Chickpea and Spinach Stew
- Quinoa and Roasted Vegetable Bowl
- Sweet Potato and Lentil Soup
- Roasted Veggie Tacos
- Baked Tofu and Vegetable Skewers
- Roasted Sweet Potato and Quinoa Bowl
- Vegetable and Chickpea Stir-Fry
- Baked Eggplant Parmesan
- Tofu and Vegetable Kebabs
- Lentil and Spinach Pasta
- Grilled Zucchini and Chickpea Salad
- Baked Sweet Potato Fries
- Vegetable and Tofu Skillet
- Roasted Carrot and Lentil Salad
- Mushroom and Spinach Stir-Fry

SNACKS

- Cucumber and Avocado Bites
- Zucchini Chips
- Carrot Sticks with Peanut Butter
- Banana Oat Energy Bites
- Coconut Chia Pudding
- Rice Cakes with Almond Butter
- Baked Kale Chips
- Roasted Chickpeas
- Stuffed Mini Bell Peppers
- Apple Slices with Sunflower Seed Butter
- Crispy Baked Tofu Cubes
- Cucumber Roll-Ups with Cream Cheese
- Chia Seed Crackers
- Roasted Pumpkin Seeds
- Strawberry Coconut Bites
- Oatmeal Snack Bars
- Crispy Roasted Kale
- Blueberry Almond Parfait
- Sesame Seed Crackers

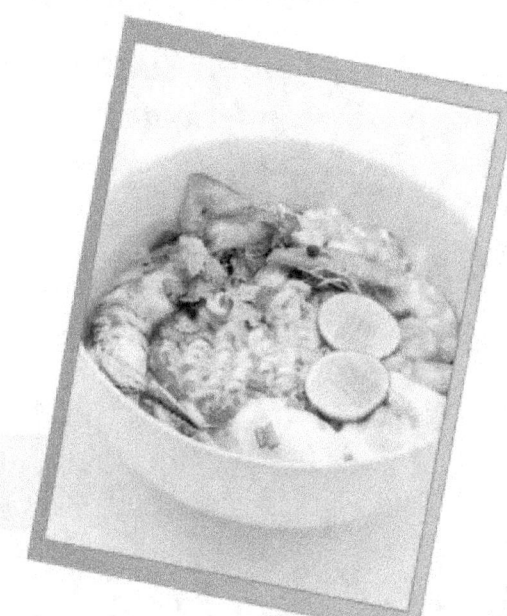

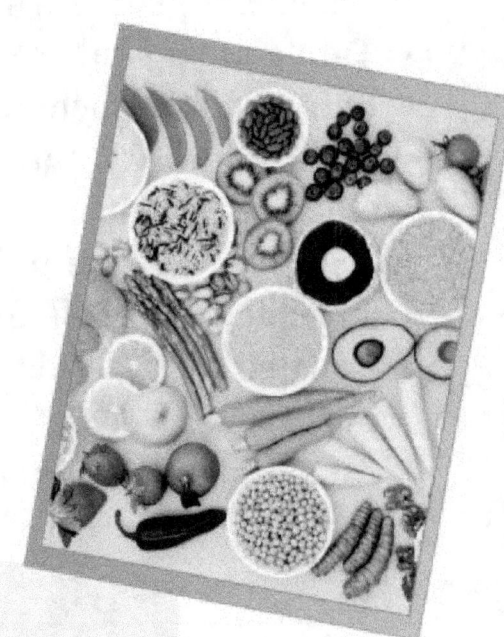

INTRODUCTION

Fast IBS Relief and Digestive Health with the Low FODMAP Vegetarian Diet

Living with digestive disorders like Irritable Bowel Syndrome (IBS) can be challenging, especially when symptoms strike without warning. Relief often seems elusive, but for those struggling with IBS and other digestive disorders, finding the right diet is crucial.

The Low FODMAP diet has emerged as an effective solution for managing these symptoms. Originally developed by researchers at Monash University, this diet focuses on reducing the intake of certain types of fermentable carbohydrates (FODMAPs) that can trigger bloating, gas, and discomfort.

For vegetarians, navigating this diet can be tricky, as many plant-based foods are high in FODMAPs, but with careful planning, it's possible to create nutritious and delicious meals that support digestive health.

Mrs. Eliza, a 70-year-old retired teacher, had always prided herself on her healthy eating habits. But after a lifetime of enjoying fruits, vegetables, and grains, she started experiencing painful bloating and stomach cramps. Diagnosed with IBS, Eliza was overwhelmed by the idea of limiting her favorite foods. However, after learning about the Low FODMAP diet for vegetarians, she decided to give it a try. She swapped her daily lentil soup for quinoa salads, replaced garlic with garlic-infused oil, and began incorporating nutrient-rich, low-FODMAP snacks like chia pudding and zucchini fritters into her routine.

In just a few weeks, Eliza found herself feeling lighter, her symptoms drastically reduced, and her energy restored. The Low FODMAP diet gave her the relief she had been seeking, proving that the right diet could truly transform her digestive health.

This guide will take you through essential tips and recipes to help you manage IBS and other digestive disorders with a vegetarian Low FODMAP approach, just like Mrs. Eliza.

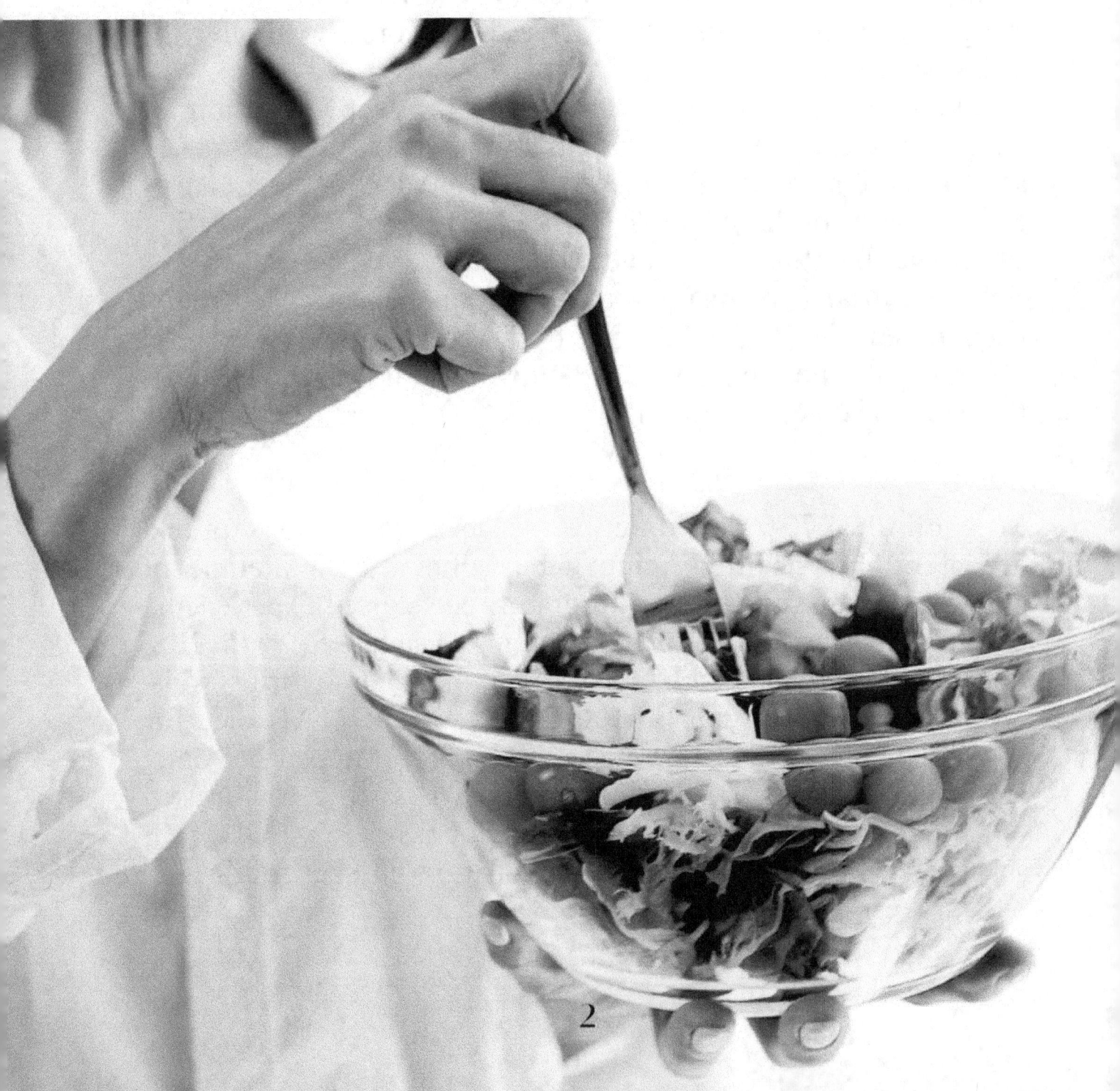

CHAPTER ONE

UNDERSTANDING THE LOW FODMAP DIET

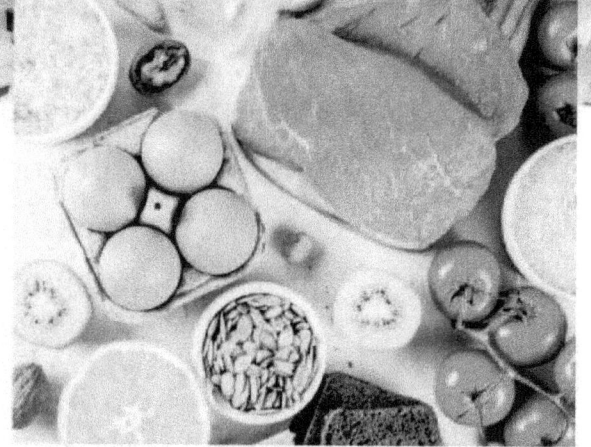

The Low FODMAP Diet is a specialized dietary plan designed to help individuals manage symptoms of irritable bowel syndrome (IBS) and other gastrointestinal conditions. FODMAP stands for fermentable oligosaccharides, disaccharides, monosaccharides, and polyols, which are short-chain carbohydrates that are poorly absorbed in the small intestine. When these carbohydrates are not fully absorbed, they travel to the large intestine, where they are fermented by gut bacteria, often leading to symptoms like bloating, gas, diarrhea, and abdominal pain.

The Low FODMAP Diet is typically divided into three phases: elimination, reintroduction, and personalization. During the elimination phase, all high-FODMAP foods are avoided to reduce symptoms. Common high-FODMAP foods include certain fruits (like apples and cherries), vegetables (such as onions and garlic), legumes, wheat-based products, dairy, and sweeteners like honey. After symptoms improve, foods are reintroduced in the reintroduction phase to identify which specific FODMAPs trigger symptoms. The final phase is personalization, where a long-term diet plan is developed based on individual tolerance levels.

For vegetarians, following the Low FODMAP Diet presents unique challenges, particularly because many vegetarian staples, such as legumes, beans, and some vegetables, are high in FODMAPs. These foods are important sources of protein and fiber in a vegetarian diet, making it crucial to find suitable low-FODMAP alternatives.

Vegetarian-friendly low-FODMAP protein sources include firm tofu, tempeh, quinoa, and certain nuts and seeds. It's also essential to be mindful of portion sizes, as some foods are only low-FODMAP in small amounts. For example, lentils and chickpeas can be consumed in small quantities if canned, as the canning process reduces their FODMAP content.

Vegetarian low-FODMAP dieters should also focus on incorporating low-FODMAP vegetables such as spinach, carrots, zucchini, and bell peppers, while avoiding high-FODMAP options like cauliflower and mushrooms. Fruits such as strawberries, oranges, and blueberries are also generally safe to eat in moderation.

By carefully selecting low-FODMAP plant-based foods, vegetarians can successfully follow the Low FODMAP Diet and manage their IBS symptoms while still maintaining a nutritious and balanced diet. Consulting a dietitian knowledgeable in both vegetarianism and FODMAPs can help ensure that all nutritional needs are met while avoiding symptom-triggering foods.

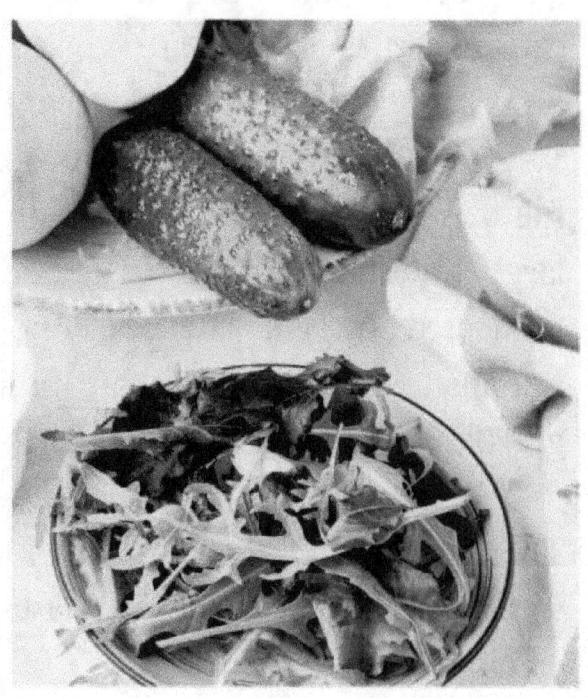

BENEFITS AND GOALS

The benefits and goals of the Low FODMAP Diet, particularly for individuals with IBS or other gastrointestinal issues, focus on improving digestive health and overall quality of life. Let's explore both:

Benefits of the Low FODMAP Diet

Symptom Relief: The primary benefit of the Low FODMAP Diet is the significant reduction in common IBS symptoms, such as bloating, abdominal pain, diarrhea, constipation, and gas. Studies show that up to 75% of IBS sufferers experience symptom relief after following this diet.

Better Gut Health: By identifying and eliminating foods that are difficult to digest, individuals can reduce irritation and inflammation in the gut, promoting better overall digestive health.

Improved Nutrient Absorption: The diet helps alleviate gastrointestinal issues that interfere with proper nutrient absorption. By managing symptoms like diarrhea, the body can absorb nutrients from food more efficiently.

Personalized Approach: After the reintroduction phase, individuals gain a clearer understanding of their specific food triggers, which allows them to tailor their diet without unnecessarily avoiding a wide range of foods.

Improved Quality of Life: The reduction in painful and uncomfortable symptoms can significantly improve daily life, enhancing physical comfort, mental well-being, and overall lifestyle satisfaction.

More Dietary Flexibility Long-Term: After successfully completing the diet's three phases, individuals can reintroduce foods that don't cause symptoms, leading to a more balanced and varied diet over time compared to the initial elimination phase.

Goals of the Low FODMAP Diet

Reduce IBS Symptoms: The primary goal is to manage and reduce symptoms associated with IBS and other functional gastrointestinal disorders. By eliminating FODMAP-rich foods, the diet minimizes the fermentation of carbohydrates in the gut, which leads to fewer digestive issues.

Identify Food Triggers: The reintroduction phase allows individuals to pinpoint specific FODMAPs that trigger their symptoms, leading to a better understanding of what their body can and cannot tolerate.

Promote Gut Comfort and Function: By avoiding high-FODMAP foods that lead to bloating and discomfort, the diet aims to improve overall gut function, reduce inflammation, and maintain a stable digestive system.

Create a Sustainable, Long-Term Eating Plan: The final goal is to develop a personalized, sustainable diet that balances symptom control with nutritional adequacy, ensuring individuals can enjoy a wide range of foods without triggering gastrointestinal distress.

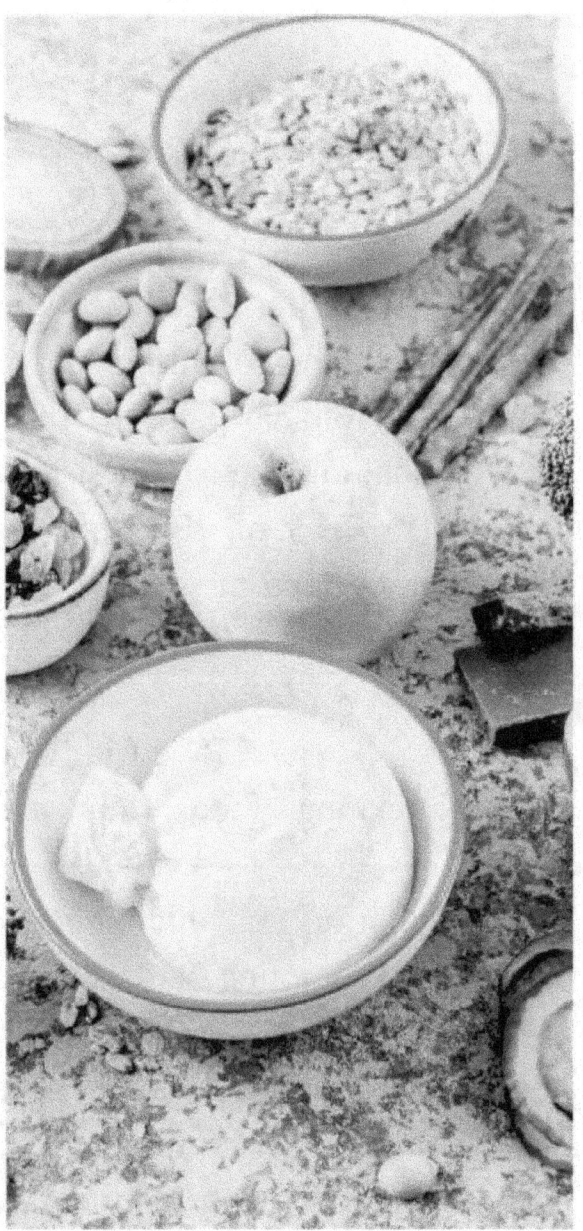

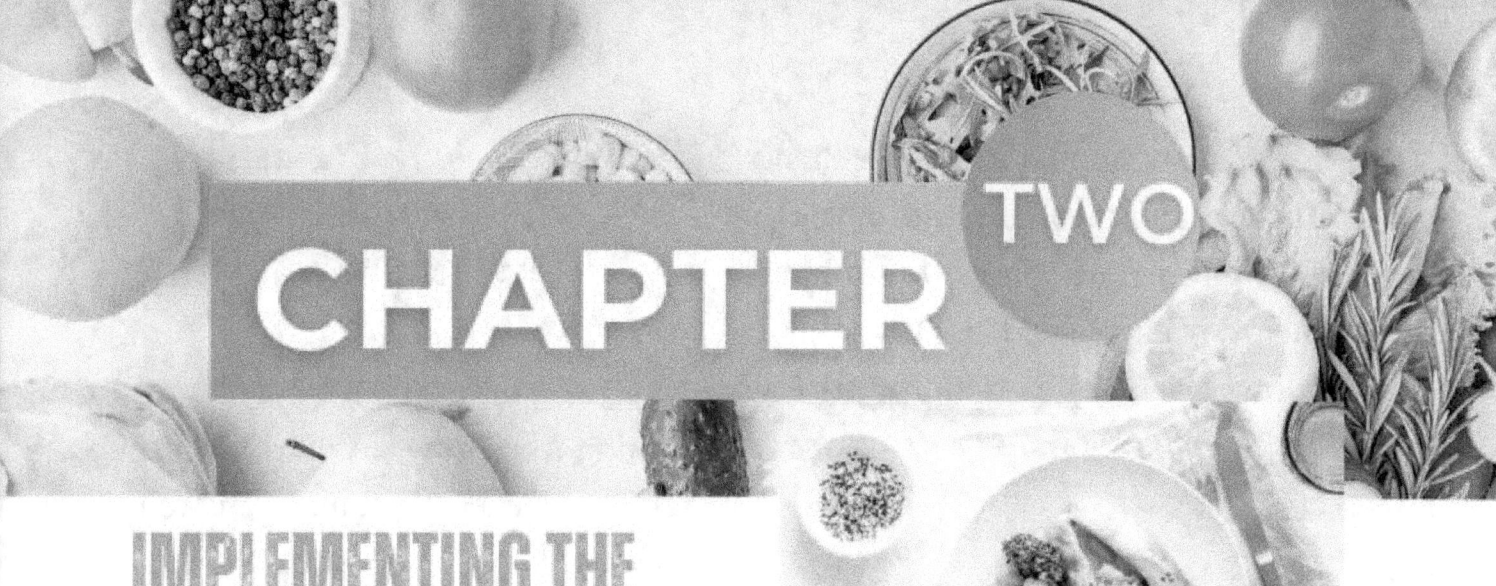

CHAPTER TWO

IMPLEMENTING THE LOW FODMAP DIET

Implementing the Low FODMAP Diet involves a structured, three-phase approach designed to manage IBS symptoms and identify food triggers. The process starts with the elimination phase, which typically lasts 4-6 weeks. During this phase, individuals avoid all high-FODMAP foods, which are known to cause digestive distress. These foods include certain fruits (like apples, pears, and stone fruits), vegetables (such as onions, garlic, and cauliflower), dairy products containing lactose, legumes, wheat-based products, and artificial sweeteners. It's essential to carefully read labels and consult with a dietitian to ensure you're following the diet correctly and receiving adequate nutrition.

Once symptoms improve, the reintroduction phase begins. During this phase, high-FODMAP foods are slowly reintroduced one at a time to determine individual tolerance. Each food or FODMAP group is introduced in small portions over several days, allowing time to observe any recurrence of symptoms. This phase is crucial for identifying specific triggers while avoiding unnecessary food restrictions.

After identifying personal food triggers, the final phase is personalization. In this phase, individuals reintroduce low-FODMAP foods that were well tolerated during the reintroduction phase and develop a long-term eating plan tailored to their specific needs. This phase allows for greater dietary variety while maintaining symptom control.

Throughout implementation, it is essential to work with a healthcare professional, especially a dietitian knowledgeable in the Low FODMAP Diet, to ensure nutritional adequacy, especially for those with dietary restrictions like vegetarians or vegans. They can help design meal plans, suggest safe alternatives, and ensure that nutrient needs are met while following the diet.

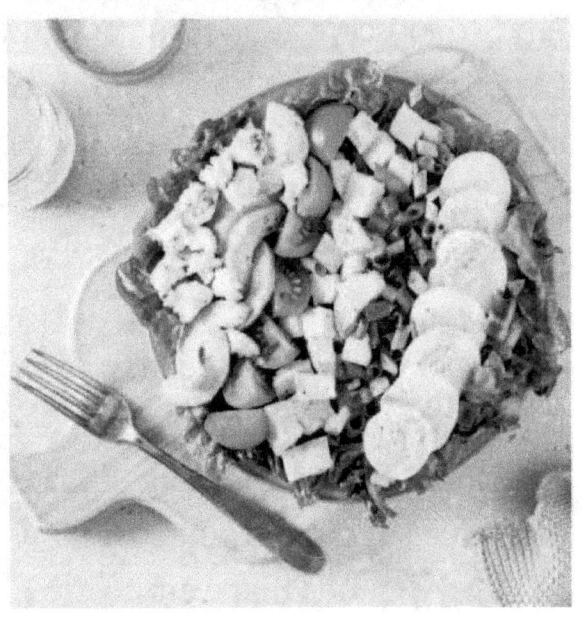

PUTTING THE LOW FODMAP DIET INTO PRACTICE

Putting the Low FODMAP Diet into practice requires careful planning, preparation, and commitment to each phase of the diet. The process starts with understanding which foods to avoid and which are safe to eat, followed by making practical adjustments in everyday life.

Step 1: Educate Yourself and Plan

Before starting the diet, familiarize yourself with high and low FODMAP foods. Many fruits, vegetables, dairy products, grains, and sweeteners contain FODMAPs, so it's essential to understand what you can and cannot eat during the elimination phase. Resources like FODMAP-friendly food lists, recipe guides, and mobile apps can help you identify safe foods.

Step 2: Phase 1 – Elimination

During the elimination phase, remove all high-FODMAP

foods from your diet for 4-6 weeks. Focus on whole foods that are naturally low in FODMAPs, such as:

Proteins: Eggs, firm tofu, and lean meats (if not vegetarian)
Vegetables: Carrots, spinach, zucchini, and bell peppers
Fruits: Bananas, strawberries, oranges, and grapes
Grains: Quinoa, rice, and oats
Ensure you're still consuming a balanced diet by incorporating low-FODMAP alternatives like lactose-free milk or almond milk, and gluten-free grains.

Step 3: Phase 2 – Reintroduction

Once your symptoms improve, start the reintroduction phase. Reintroduce one high-FODMAP food at a time, like apples or garlic, in small portions. Pay close attention to your body's reactions, recording any symptoms to identify which FODMAPs you tolerate well and which ones trigger issues.

Step 4: Phase 3 – Personalization

In the personalization phase, create a long-term diet based on what you've learned. Reintroduce tolerable foods and continue avoiding problematic FODMAPs. This tailored approach ensures you have a varied, nutritionally balanced diet without triggering symptoms.

Tips for Success:

Meal Planning: Plan meals ahead of time to ensure you have low-FODMAP options on hand.
Label Reading: Be diligent about checking food labels for hidden FODMAP ingredients, especially in processed foods.

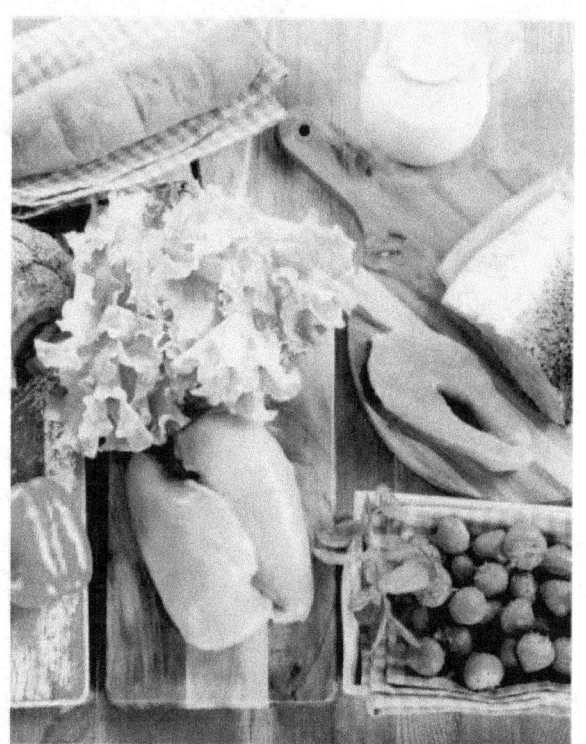

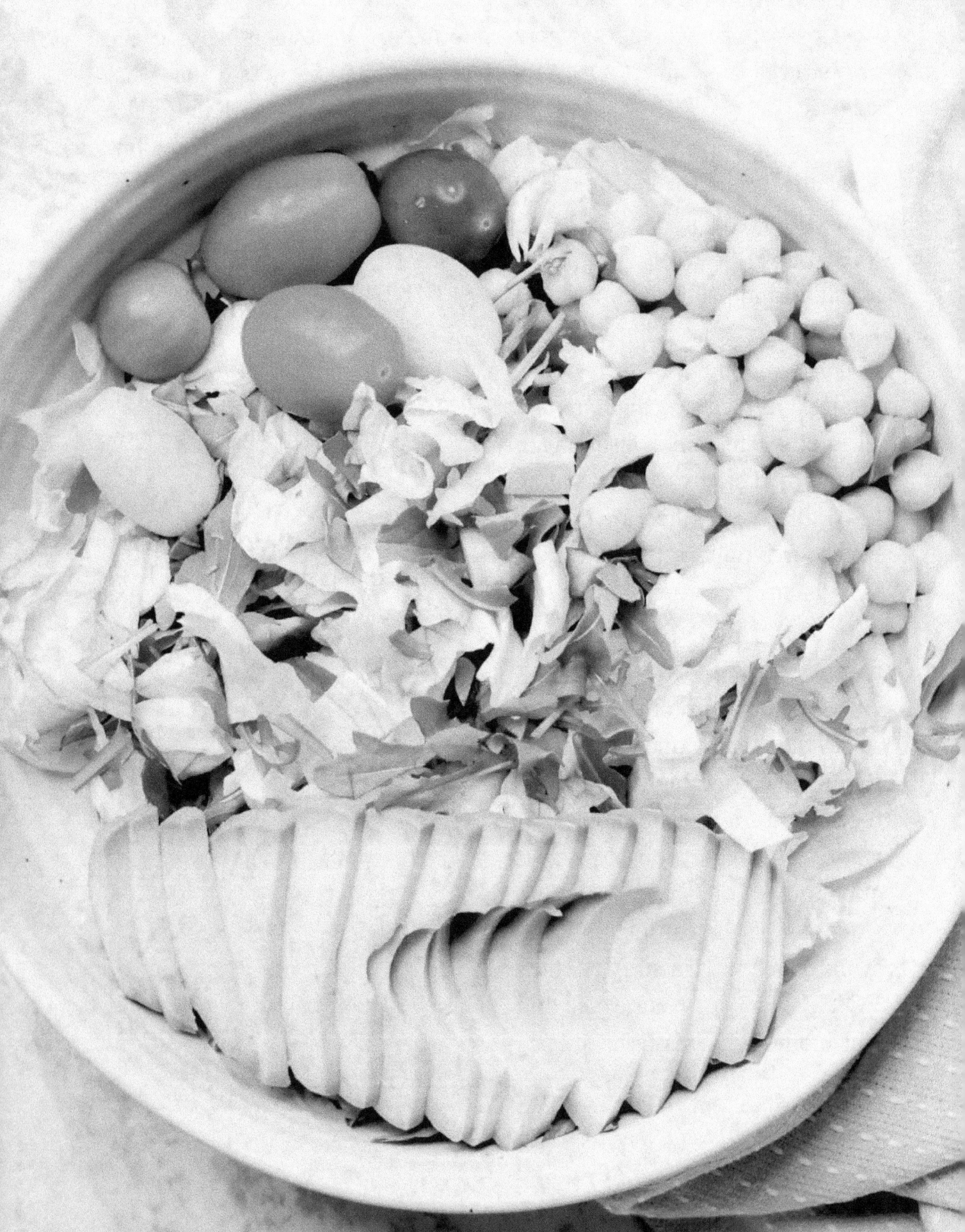

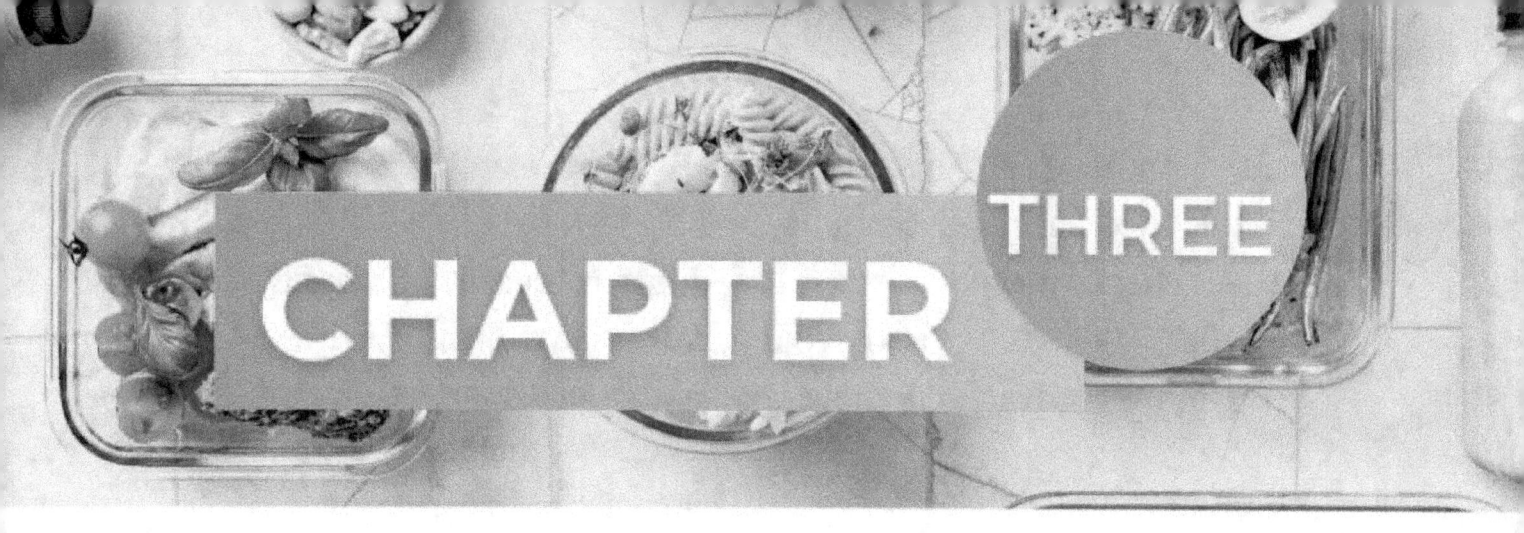

CHAPTER THREE

LOW FODMAP LIFESTYLE AND DIGESTIVE HEALTH TIPS

Adopting a Low FODMAP lifestyle can significantly improve digestive health, especially for individuals with IBS or other gastrointestinal disorders. This approach emphasizes managing symptoms while incorporating long-term healthy habits. Here are some tips to integrate the Low FODMAP diet into your lifestyle and promote better digestive health:

1. Meal Planning and Preparation

Plan your meals and snacks ahead of time to avoid accidentally consuming high-FODMAP foods. Focus on simple, whole foods that are naturally low in FODMAPs, such as lean proteins, rice, and low-FODMAP fruits and vegetables.

Batch-cooking and storing meals can help you stick to the diet, especially during busy days.

2. Read Labels Carefully

Processed foods often contain hidden high-FODMAP ingredients like high-fructose corn syrup, honey, or onion powder. Make it a habit to read food labels thoroughly to ensure you're avoiding these ingredients. Many FODMAP-friendly apps can help you identify safe foods.

3. Portion Control

Some foods are low in FODMAPs only in smaller portions. For instance, certain legumes and fruits may be well tolerated in small amounts. Always check serving sizes for low-FODMAP options and avoid overeating them to prevent symptoms.

4. Stay Hydrated

Drinking plenty of water throughout the day supports digestive health and helps prevent constipation, a common issue for those with IBS. Avoid carbonated drinks and excessive caffeine, as they can aggravate bloating and gas.

5. Mindful Eating

Practicing mindful eating can enhance digestion. Chew your food slowly and thoroughly, and eat in a calm environment. This allows the digestive system to process food more efficiently and reduces the likelihood of symptoms like bloating or discomfort.

6. Incorporate Low-FODMAP Fiber

Fiber is crucial for digestive health, but many high-FODMAP foods, like beans and lentils, are rich in fiber. To maintain adequate fiber intake, choose low-FODMAP sources such as oats, chia seeds, flaxseeds, and zucchini. Gradually increase your fiber intake to avoid overwhelming your digestive system.

7. Manage Stress

Stress can exacerbate IBS symptoms. Incorporate stress-reducing activities into your daily routine, such as yoga, meditation, or deep breathing exercises. Managing stress improves digestion and overall well-being.

8. Probiotics and Gut Health

Consider adding probiotics to your routine, as they promote healthy gut bacteria. Certain strains of probiotics may improve gut health and help alleviate IBS symptoms. Always consult with a healthcare provider before introducing supplements into your diet.

9. Keep a Food Diary

Tracking your meals and symptoms in a food diary can help identify any patterns or triggers, making it easier to personalize your Low FODMAP diet. Recording what you eat, how much, and when symptoms occur provides valuable insight into managing your digestive health.

10. Seek Professional Guidance

A dietitian experienced in the Low FODMAP diet can provide tailored advice, ensuring you meet nutritional needs while avoiding FODMAP triggers. They can also help adjust the diet for long-term sustainability.

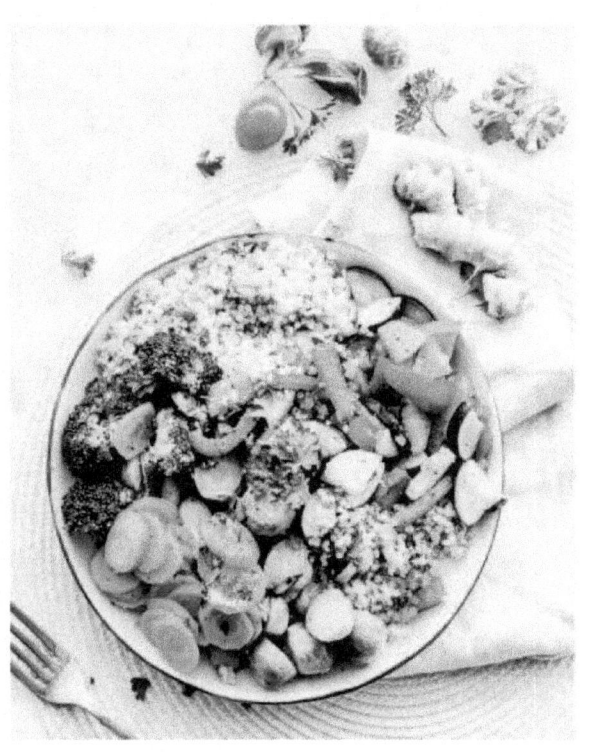

COOKING TIPS AND MODIFICATION

Cooking on a Low FODMAP diet can be challenging for vegetarians, as many common vegetarian protein sources, such as beans and lentils, are high in FODMAPs. However, with a few cooking tips and modifications, it's possible to create satisfying, nutrient-rich meals while adhering to the diet.

1. Use Low-FODMAP Protein Sources

Vegetarian proteins like tofu (firm and drained), tempeh, quinoa, and small servings of canned lentils and chickpeas are excellent substitutes for high-FODMAP legumes. Canned legumes are lower in FODMAPs due to the draining process, so be sure to rinse them thoroughly before use.

2. Replace Garlic and Onion

Garlic and onions, staples in many vegetarian recipes, are high in FODMAPs. However, their flavors can still be achieved using low-FODMAP alternatives. Garlic-infused oil is a great option, as the FODMAPs do not dissolve in oil, making it safe to consume. For onions, use the green tops of scallions or chives to add a similar flavor without triggering symptoms.

3. Choose Low-FODMAP Vegetables

Opt for low-FODMAP vegetables like carrots, spinach, bell peppers, zucchini, and eggplant. These can be roasted, grilled, or sautéed for flavorful dishes. Avoid high-FODMAP vegetables like broccoli, cauliflower, and mushrooms, which may cause digestive discomfort.

4. Pay Attention to Portion Sizes

Some foods, such as almonds or sweet potatoes, are only low-FODMAP in small portions. Be mindful of how much you consume to stay within the recommended limits and avoid triggering symptoms.

5. Make Dairy-Free Substitutions

For dairy-free vegetarians, opt for lactose-free milk, almond milk, or rice milk, which are all low-FODMAP alternatives. When cooking, use these substitutions in sauces, smoothies, or baked goods.

By applying these cooking tips and modifications, vegetarians can enjoy a balanced, satisfying Low FODMAP diet without sacrificing flavor or nutrition.

Breakfast Recipes

HERE ARE SIMPLE, LOW FODMAP BREAKFAST RECIPES, EACH WITH ITS INGREDIENTS, DIRECTIONS, NUTRITIONAL INFORMATION, SERVINGS, AND COOKING TIME.

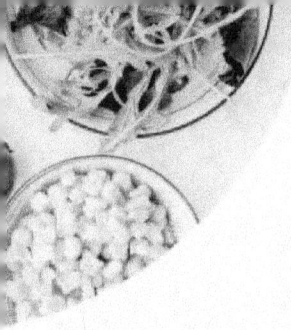

BANANA OAT
PANCAKES

INGREDIENTS

- 1 ripe banana
- 1 cup rolled oats (gluten-free)
- 1/2 cup almond milk (unsweetened)
- 1/2 tsp baking powder
- 1 tsp vanilla extract
- 1/2 tsp cinnamon

DIRECTIONS

1. Blend all ingredients in a blender until smooth.
2. Heat a non-stick pan over medium heat.
3. Pour batter into small pancake circles.
4. Cook for 2-3 minutes on each side until golden brown.
5. Serve with maple syrup or fresh low-FODMAP fruits.
6. Enjoy warm.

More Info :

Nutrition per Serving:
Calories: 290
Protein: 7g
Carbs: 50g
Fiber: 6g
Servings: 2
Cooking Time: 15 minutes

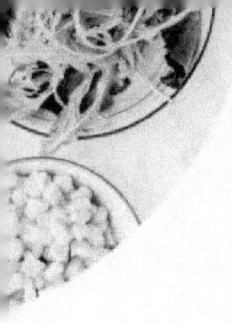

TOFU
SCRAMBLE

INGREDIENTS

- /2 block firm tofu (drained)
- 1/2 tsp turmeric
- 1 tbsp olive oil
- 1/4 cup chopped spinach
- 1/4 cup diced red bell pepper
- Salt and pepper to taste

DIRECTIONS

1. Heat oil in a pan over medium heat.
2. Crumble tofu into the pan.
3. Add turmeric, salt, and pepper; stir well.
4. Toss in spinach and bell pepper, sauté for 3-4 minutes.
5. Cook until tofu is golden and veggies are tender.
6. Serve immediately.

More Info :

Nutrition per Serving:
Calories: 240
Protein: 12g
Carbs: 8g
Fiber: 4g
Servings: 1-2
Cooking Time: 10 minutes

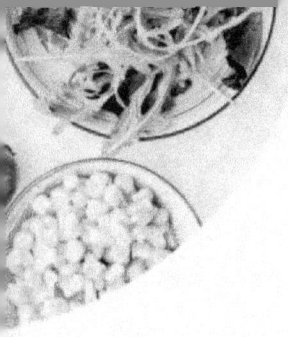

CHIA PUDDING

INGREDIENTS

- 3 tbsp chia seeds
- 1 cup almond milk (unsweetened)
- 1 tsp vanilla extract
- 1 tbsp maple syrup

DIRECTIONS

1. Combine chia seeds, almond milk, vanilla, and maple syrup in a bowl.
2. Stir well to avoid clumping.
3. Refrigerate for at least 4 hours or overnight.
4. Stir again before serving.
5. Top with low-FODMAP fruits like strawberries.
6. Enjoy chilled.

More Info :

Nutrition per Serving:
Calories: 180
Protein: 6g
Fiber: 12g
Omega-3: 4g
Servings: 2
Cooking Time: 5 minutes (plus refrigeration)

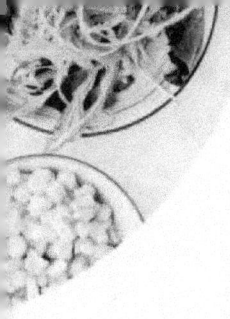

QUINOA PORRIDGE

INGREDIENTS

- 1/2 cup quinoa
- 1 cup almond milk (unsweetened)
- 1 tsp maple syrup
- 1/2 tsp cinnamon
- 1/4 cup blueberries

DIRECTIONS

1. Rinse quinoa under cold water.
2. In a pot, combine quinoa, almond milk, and cinnamon.
3. Bring to a boil, then simmer for 15 minutes.
4. Stir in maple syrup and cook until quinoa is tender.
5. Top with fresh blueberries.
6. Serve warm.

More Info :

Nutrition per Serving:
Calories: 260
Protein: 8g
Carbs: 45g
Fiber: 5g
Servings: 2
Cooking Time: 20 minutes

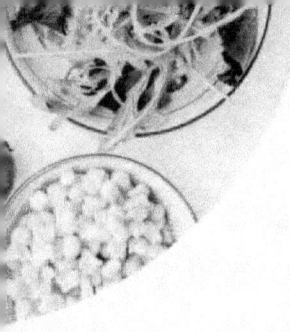

SMOOTHIE BOWL

INGREDIENTS

- 1/2 cup frozen strawberries
- 1/2 frozen banana
- 1/2 cup almond milk (unsweetened)
- 2 tbsp chia seeds
- 1/4 cup gluten-free granola

DIRECTIONS

1. Blend strawberries, banana, and almond milk until smooth.
2. Pour into a bowl.
3. Top with chia seeds and granola.
4. Add additional low-FODMAP fruits if desired.
5. Serve chilled.
6. Enjoy immediately.

More Info :

Nutrition per Serving:
Calories: 320
Protein: 6g
Carbs: 50g
Fiber: 10g
Servings: 1
Cooking Time: 5 minutes

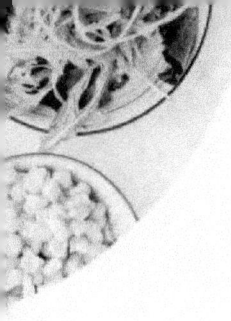

ZUCCHINI FRITTERS

INGREDIENTS

- 1 medium zucchini (grated)
- 1/4 cup gluten-free flour
- 1 egg
- 1 tbsp olive oil
- Salt and pepper to taste

DIRECTIONS

1. Squeeze excess water from grated zucchini.
2. Mix zucchini, flour, egg, salt, and pepper in a bowl.
3. Heat oil in a pan over medium heat.
4. Spoon mixture into the pan, flattening into fritters.
5. Cook 3-4 minutes per side until golden brown.
6. Serve hot.

More Info :

Nutrition per Serving:
Calories: 180
Protein: 6g
Carbs: 18g
Fiber: 2g
Servings: 2
Cooking Time: 15 minutes

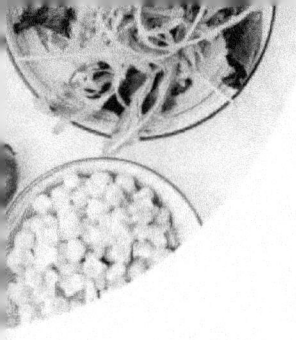

COCONUT YOGURT WITH BERRIES

INGREDIENTS

- 1/2 cup coconut yogurt (unsweetened)
- 1/4 cup strawberries (sliced)
- 1 tbsp chia seeds
- 1 tbsp maple syrup

DIRECTIONS

1. In a bowl, mix coconut yogurt and maple syrup.
2. Top with strawberries and chia seeds.
3. Stir well or layer the ingredients.
4. Serve immediately.
5. Enjoy as a light, fresh breakfast.
6. Optional: Add gluten-free granola.

More Info :

Nutrition per Serving:
Calories: 210
Protein: 3g
Fiber: 5g
Healthy Fats: 9g
Servings: 1
Cooking Time: 5 minutes

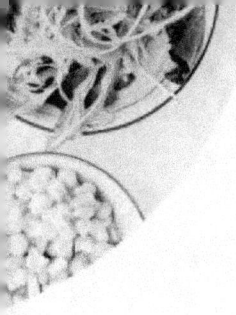

PUMPKIN OATMEAL

INGREDIENTS

- 1/2 cup gluten-free rolled oats
- 1 cup almond milk (unsweetened)
- 1/4 cup canned pumpkin (unsweetened)
- 1/2 tsp cinnamon
- 1 tbsp maple syrup

DIRECTIONS

1. In a pot, combine oats and almond milk.
2. Bring to a simmer and cook until oats soften.
3. Stir in pumpkin, cinnamon, and maple syrup.
4. Cook for another 2-3 minutes.
5. Serve warm with additional cinnamon if desired.

More Info :

Nutrition per Serving:
Calories: 240
Protein: 6g
Carbs: 42g
Fiber: 6g
Servings: 2
Cooking Time: 10 minutes

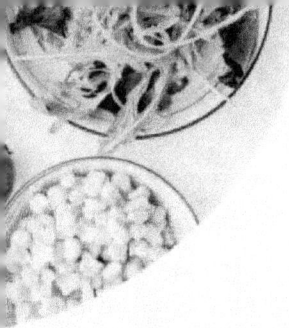

AVOCADO TOAST

INGREDIENTS

- 1 ripe avocado
- 2 slices gluten-free bread
- 1 tsp lemon juice
- Salt and pepper to taste
- 1 tbsp olive oil

DIRECTIONS

1. Toast the gluten-free bread until crispy.
2. Mash avocado in a bowl with lemon juice, salt, and pepper.
3. Spread avocado mixture onto toast.
4. Drizzle with olive oil.
5. Serve immediately.
6. Enjoy as a quick, savory breakfast.

More Info :

Nutrition per Serving:
Calories: 300
Protein: 4g
Healthy Fats: 21g
Fiber: 8g
Servings: 1-2
Cooking Time: 5 minutes

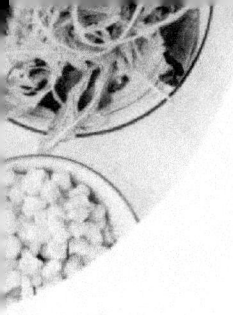

BUCKWHEAT PANCAKES

INGREDIENTS

- 1/2 cup buckwheat flour
- 1/2 cup almond milk (unsweetened)
- 1 egg
- 1 tbsp maple syrup
- 1/2 tsp baking powder

DIRECTIONS

1. Mix buckwheat flour, almond milk, egg, and baking powder.
2. Heat a non-stick pan over medium heat.
3. Pour batter into small pancake circles.
4. Cook for 2-3 minutes on each side.
5. Drizzle with maple syrup or top with low-FODMAP fruits.
6. Serve warm.

More Info :

Nutrition per Serving:
Calories: 250
Protein: 8g
Carbs: 35g
Fiber: 5g
Servings: 2
Cooking Time: 15 minutes

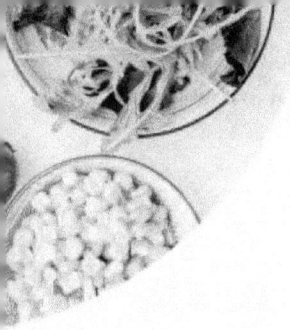

POLENTA PORRIDGE

INGREDIENTS

- 1/2 cup polenta
- 1 1/2 cups almond milk (unsweetened)
- 1 tbsp maple syrup
- 1/2 tsp cinnamon
- 1/4 cup blueberries

DIRECTIONS

1. In a pot, combine polenta and almond milk.
2. Bring to a boil, then simmer for 10-15 minutes, stirring occasionally.
3. Add maple syrup and cinnamon, stirring well.
4. Cook until thick and creamy.
5. Top with blueberries before serving.
6. Serve warm.

More Info :

Nutrition per Serving:
Calories: 250
Protein: 6g
Carbs: 44g
Fiber: 5g
Servings: 2
Cooking Time: 15 minutes

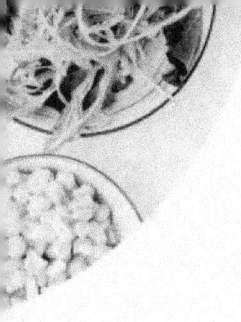

SWEET POTATO BREAKFAST HASH

INGREDIENTS

- 1 medium sweet potato (diced)
- 1 tbsp olive oil
- 1/4 cup red bell pepper (diced)
- 1/4 cup spinach (chopped)
- Salt and pepper to taste

DIRECTIONS

1. Heat olive oil in a pan over medium heat.
2. Add diced sweet potato and cook for 10-12 minutes until soft.
3. Add bell pepper and spinach, cooking for another 3-4 minutes.
4. Season with salt and pepper.
5. Serve immediately as a hearty breakfast.

More Info :

Nutrition per Serving:
Calories: 180
Protein: 2g
Carbs: 30g
Fiber: 5g
Servings: 1-2
Cooking Time: 15 minutes

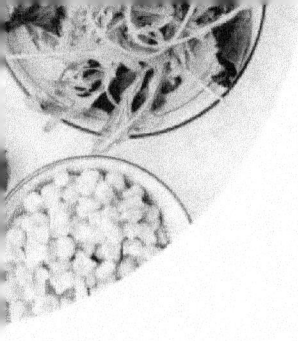

EGGPLANT BREAKFAST WRAP

INGREDIENTS

- 1/2 cup roasted eggplant (sliced)
- 2 gluten-free tortillas
- 1/4 cup spinach
- 2 tbsp hummus (low FODMAP)
- Salt and pepper to taste

DIRECTIONS

1. Spread hummus on the gluten-free tortillas.
2. Add roasted eggplant slices and spinach.
3. Season with salt and pepper.
4. Roll up the tortilla into a wrap.
5. Serve warm or chilled.
6. Enjoy as a quick, on-the-go breakfast.

More Info :

Nutrition per Serving:
Calories: 220
Protein: 5g
Carbs: 38g
Fiber: 6g
Servings: 1-2
Cooking Time: 10 minutes

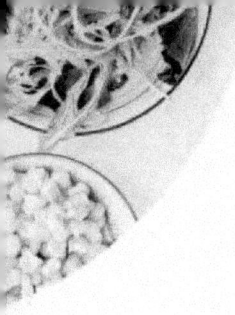

PEANUT BUTTER CHIA TOAST

INGREDIENTS

- 2 slices gluten-free bread
- 2 tbsp peanut butter (unsweetened)
- 1 tsp chia seeds
- 1/2 banana (sliced)

DIRECTIONS

1. Toast the gluten-free bread until crispy.
2. Spread peanut butter evenly on each slice.
3. Top with chia seeds and banana slices.
4. Serve immediately for a nutrient-packed breakfast.

More Info :

Nutrition per Serving:
Calories: 340
Protein: 12g
Carbs: 40g
Fiber: 8g
Servings: 1-2
Cooking Time: 5 minutes

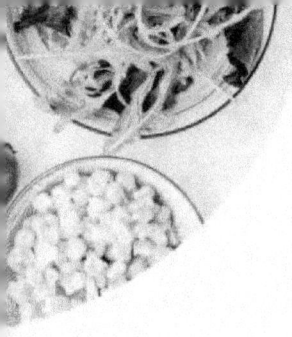

BERRY COCONUT
SMOOTHIE

INGREDIENTS

- 1/2 cup frozen strawberries
- 1/2 cup coconut milk (unsweetened)
- 1/4 cup blueberries
- 1 tbsp chia seeds
- 1 tbsp maple syrup

DIRECTIONS

1. Blend strawberries, blueberries, coconut milk, and maple syrup until smooth.
2. Pour into a glass.
3. Stir in chia seeds.
4. Serve chilled.
5. Enjoy as a refreshing breakfast smoothie.

More Info :

Nutrition per Serving:
Calories: 200
Protein: 3g
Carbs: 25g
Fiber: 6g
Servings: 1
Cooking Time: 5 minutes

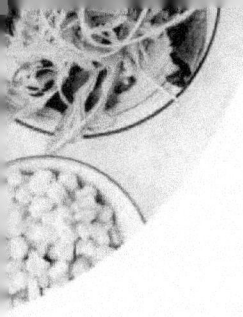

BUCKWHEAT PORRIDGE

INGREDIENTS

- 1/2 cup buckwheat groats
- 1 cup almond milk (unsweetened)
- 1 tsp maple syrup
- 1/2 tsp cinnamon
- 1/4 cup strawberries (sliced)

DIRECTIONS

1. In a pot, combine buckwheat and almond milk.
2. Bring to a boil, then simmer for 10-12 minutes until soft.
3. Stir in maple syrup and cinnamon.
4. Top with fresh strawberries.
5. Serve warm for a cozy breakfast.

More Info :

Nutrition per Serving:
Calories: 240
Protein: 6g
Carbs: 40g
Fiber: 5g
Servings: 2
Cooking Time: 15 minutes

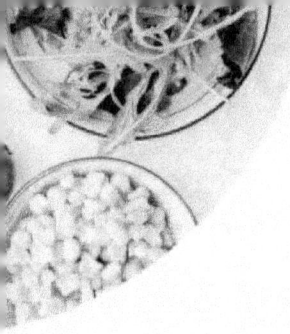

OVERNIGHT OATS

INGREDIENTS

- 1/2 cup gluten-free rolled oats
- 1/2 cup almond milk (unsweetened)
- 1 tbsp chia seeds
- 1 tsp maple syrup
- 1/4 cup blueberries

DIRECTIONS

1. In a jar, combine oats, almond milk, chia seeds, and maple syrup.
2. Stir well, cover, and refrigerate overnight.
3. In the morning, top with blueberries.
4. Serve chilled.
5. Enjoy as a make-ahead breakfast.

More Info :

Nutrition per Serving:
Calories: 200
Protein: 6g
Carbs: 35g
Fiber: 6g
Servings: 1
Cooking Time: 5 minutes (plus overnight)

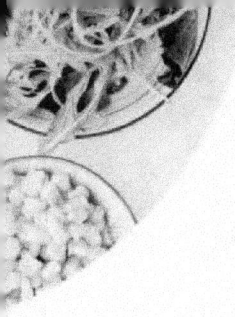

GLUTEN-FREE WAFFLES

INGREDIENTS

- 1 cup gluten-free flour
- 1/2 cup almond milk (unsweetened)
- 1 egg
- 1 tbsp maple syrup
- 1/2 tsp baking powder

DIRECTIONS

1. Mix gluten-free flour, almond milk, egg, and baking powder.
2. Preheat waffle iron.
3. Pour batter into the waffle iron and cook according to manufacturer's instructions.
4. Serve with maple syrup or low-FODMAP fruits.
5. Enjoy warm and crispy waffles.

More Info :

Nutrition per Serving:
Calories: 320
Protein: 8g
Carbs: 55g
Fiber: 3g
Servings: 2
Cooking Time: 15 minutes

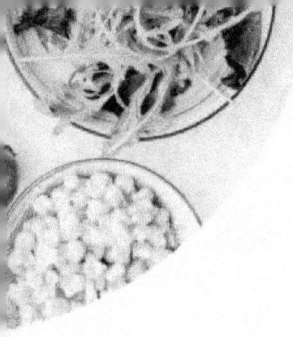

COCONUT RICE
PORRIDGE

INGREDIENTS

- 1/2 cup jasmine rice
- 1 cup coconut milk (unsweetened)
- 1 tsp maple syrup
- 1/4 tsp cinnamon
- 1/4 cup mango (diced)

DIRECTIONS

1. Cook jasmine rice according to package instructions.
2. In a pot, combine cooked rice, coconut milk, and cinnamon.
3. Heat until warmed through.
4. Stir in maple syrup and top with diced mango.
5. Serve warm for a tropical twist.

More Info :

Nutrition per Serving:
Calories: 290
Protein: 5g
Carbs: 45g
Fiber: 3g
Servings: 2
Cooking Time: 20 minutes

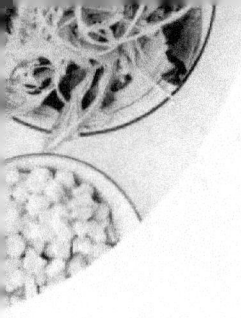

LOW-FODMAP GRANOLA

INGREDIENTS

- 2 cups gluten-free oats
- 1/4 cup shredded coconut (unsweetened)
- 1/4 cup maple syrup
- 1/4 cup sunflower seeds
- 1 tbsp coconut oil (melted)

DIRECTIONS

1. Preheat oven to 325°F (165°C).
2. In a bowl, mix oats, coconut, sunflower seeds, and melted coconut oil.
3. Add maple syrup and stir until well coated.
4. Spread on a baking sheet and bake for 20 minutes, stirring halfway through.
5. Let cool and store in an airtight container.
6. Serve with almond milk or low-FODMAP fruits.

More Info :

Nutrition per Serving:
Calories: 220
Protein: 4g
Carbs: 30g
Fiber: 5g
Servings: 6
Cooking Time: 25 minutes

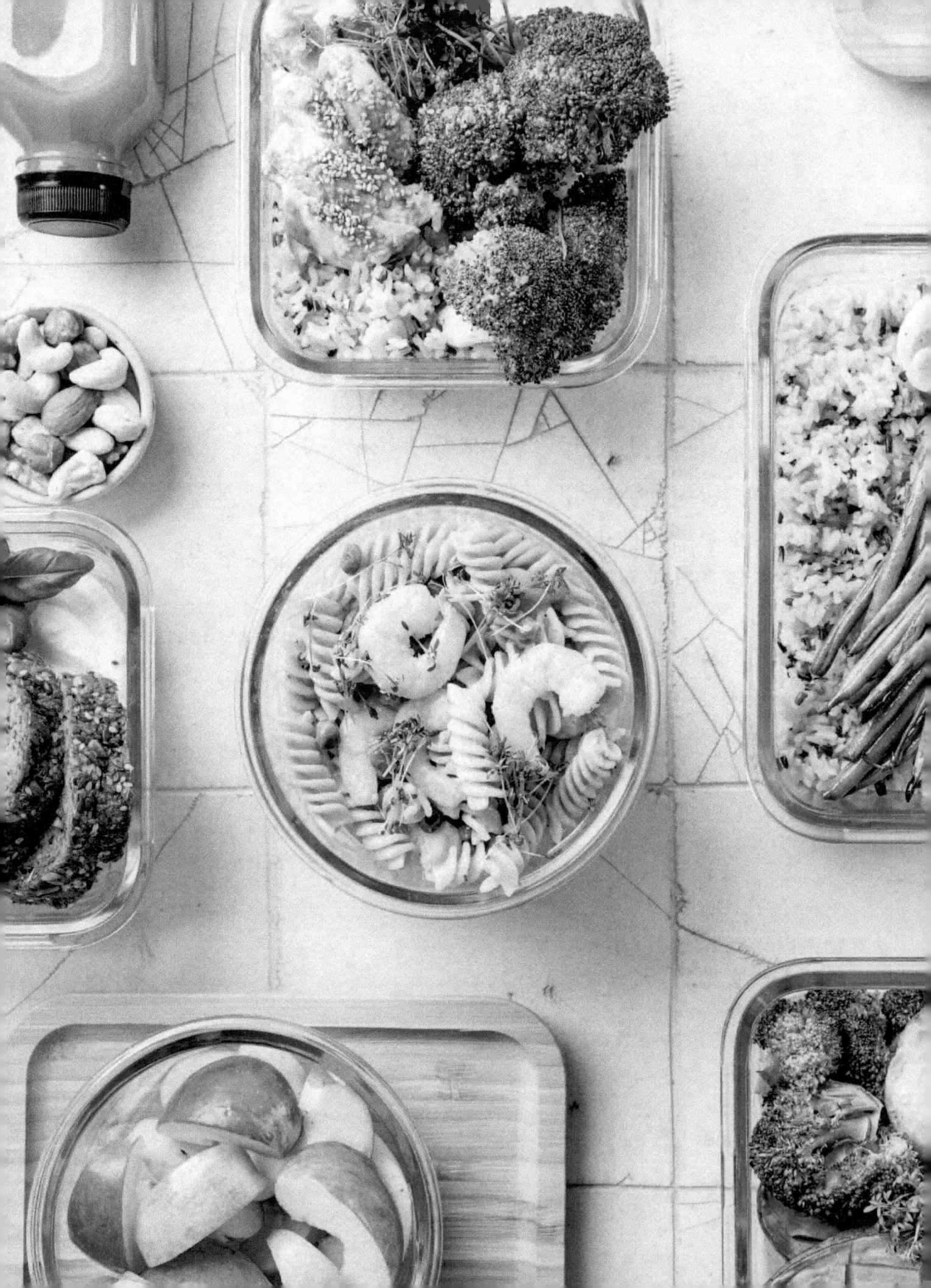

Lunch Recipes

HERE ARE SIMPLE, LOW FODMAP LUNCH RECIPES, EACH WITH ITS INGREDIENTS, DIRECTIONS, NUTRITIONAL INFORMATION, SERVINGS, AND COOKING TIME.

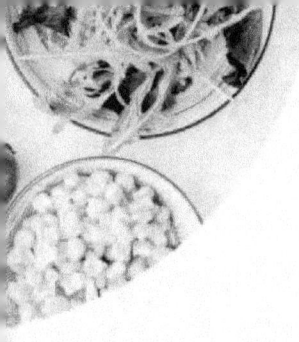

GRILLED VEGETABLE QUINOA SALAD

INGREDIENTS

- 1/2 cup quinoa
- 1 zucchini (sliced)
- 1 red bell pepper (sliced)
- 1 tbsp olive oil
- 1 tbsp lemon juice
- Salt and pepper to taste

DIRECTIONS

1. Cook quinoa according to package instructions.
2. Grill zucchini and bell pepper in olive oil until tender.
3. In a bowl, mix quinoa, grilled vegetables, and lemon juice.
4. Season with salt and pepper.
5. Serve warm or chilled.

More Info :

Nutrition per Serving:
Calories: 250
Protein: 7g
Carbs: 40g
Fiber: 6g
Servings: 2
Cooking Time: 20 minutes

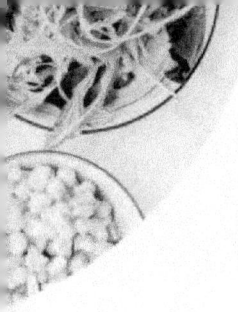

VEGETARIAN STUFFED BELL PEPPERS

INGREDIENTS

- 2 large bell peppers (halved)
- 1/2 cup cooked quinoa
- 1/4 cup canned lentils (rinsed)
- 1/4 cup diced tomatoes
- 1 tsp olive oil
- Salt and pepper to taste

DIRECTIONS

1. Preheat oven to 350°F (175°C).
2. Mix quinoa, lentils, tomatoes, and olive oil in a bowl.
3. Stuff the mixture into halved bell peppers.
4. Bake for 20 minutes until peppers are tender.
5. Season with salt and pepper.
6. Serve hot.

More Info :

Nutrition per Serving:
Calories: 230
Protein: 9g
Carbs: 45g
Fiber: 7g
Servings: 2
Cooking Time: 30 minutes

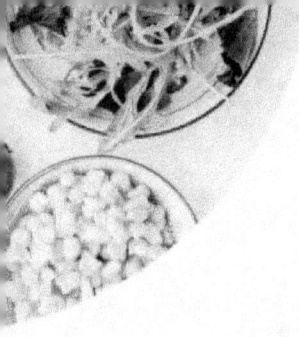

ZUCCHINI NOODLES
WITH PESTO

INGREDIENTS

- 2 medium zucchinis (spiralized into noodles)
- 1/4 cup basil pesto (low-FODMAP)
- 1 tbsp olive oil
- 1 tbsp lemon juice
- Salt and pepper to taste

DIRECTIONS

1. Heat olive oil in a pan over medium heat.
2. Add zucchini noodles and sauté for 2-3 minutes.
3. Remove from heat and toss with pesto and lemon juice.
4. Season with salt and pepper.
5. Serve immediately.
6. Enjoy a light, fresh lunch.

More Info :

Nutrition per Serving:
Calories: 180
Protein: 4g
Carbs: 15g
Fiber: 3g
Servings: 1-2
Cooking Time: 10 minutes

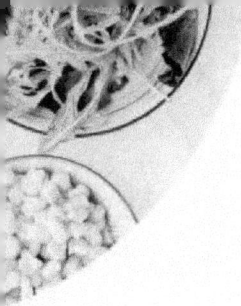

TOFU STIR-FRY WITH BOK CHOY

INGREDIENTS

- 1/2 block firm tofu (cubed)
- 1 cup bok choy (chopped)
- 1/4 cup carrots (sliced)
- 1 tbsp soy sauce (low sodium)
- 1 tbsp sesame oil
- 1 tbsp sesame seeds

DIRECTIONS

1. Heat sesame oil in a pan over medium heat.
2. Add tofu cubes and stir-fry until golden brown.
3. Add bok choy and carrots, cook for 3-4 minutes.
4. Stir in soy sauce and cook for another minute.
5. Sprinkle with sesame seeds before serving.
6. Serve hot.

More Info :

Nutrition per Serving:
Calories: 220
Protein: 11g
Carbs: 10g
Fiber: 4g
Servings: 1
Cooking Time: 15 minutes

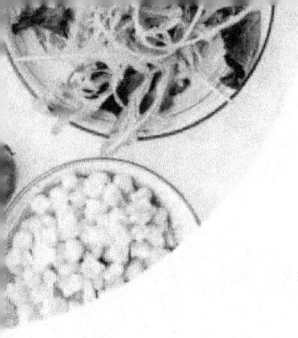

CUCUMBER AVOCADO SALAD

INGREDIENTS

- 1 cucumber (sliced)
- 1 avocado (diced)
- 1 tbsp lemon juice
- 1 tbsp olive oil
- Salt and pepper to taste

DIRECTIONS

1. In a bowl, mix cucumber and avocado.
2. Drizzle with lemon juice and olive oil.
3. Season with salt and pepper.
4. Toss gently to combine.
5. Serve immediately as a refreshing salad.

More Info :

Nutrition per Serving:
Calories: 250
Protein: 3g
Carbs: 12g
Fiber: 8g
Servings: 1-2
Cooking Time: 5 minutes

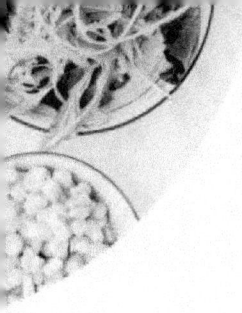

LENTIL AND SPINACH SOUP

INGREDIENTS

- 1/2 cup canned lentils (rinsed)
- 1 cup spinach (chopped)
- 2 cups vegetable broth (low-FODMAP)
- 1/4 cup carrots (diced)
- 1 tbsp olive oil

DIRECTIONS

1. Heat olive oil in a pot over medium heat.
2. Add carrots and sauté for 3 minutes.
3. Pour in vegetable broth and bring to a boil.
4. Add lentils and spinach, simmer for 10 minutes.
5. Season with salt and pepper to taste.
6. Serve hot.

More Info :

Nutrition per Serving:
Calories: 200
Protein: 9g
Carbs: 30g
Fiber: 9g
Servings: 2
Cooking Time: 20 minutes

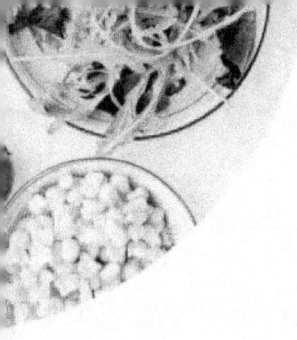

VEGETABLE STIR-FRY WITH RICE

INGREDIENTS

- 1/2 cup cooked rice
- 1/4 cup carrots (sliced)
- 1/4 cup zucchini (sliced)
- 1 tbsp soy sauce (low sodium)
- 1 tbsp olive oil

DIRECTIONS

1. Heat olive oil in a pan over medium heat.
2. Add carrots and zucchini, stir-fry for 4-5 minutes.
3. Stir in cooked rice and soy sauce.
4. Cook for another 2 minutes until well combined.
5. Serve hot and enjoy.
6. Optionally, add sesame seeds for extra flavor.

More Info :

Nutrition per Serving:
Calories: 240
Protein: 5g
Carbs: 42g
Fiber: 3g
Servings: 1
Cooking Time: 15 minutes

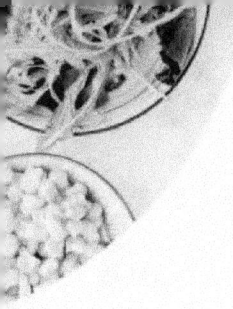

GRILLED EGGPLANT WITH CHICKPEAS

INGREDIENTS

- 1/2 eggplant (sliced)
- 1/2 cup canned chickpeas (rinsed)
- 1 tbsp olive oil
- 1 tbsp balsamic vinegar
- Salt and pepper to taste

DIRECTIONS

1. Grill eggplant slices in olive oil until tender.
2. In a bowl, toss chickpeas with balsamic vinegar, salt, and pepper.
3. Plate grilled eggplant and top with chickpeas.
4. Drizzle with more olive oil if desired.
5. Serve warm.
6. Enjoy a savory, nutritious lunch.

More Info :

Nutrition per Serving:
Calories: 260
Protein: 7g
Carbs: 30g
Fiber: 9g
Servings: 1
Cooking Time: 15 minutes

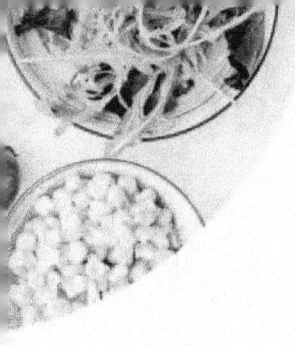

AVOCADO CHICKPEA WRAP

INGREDIENTS

- 1 gluten-free tortilla
- 1/2 avocado (mashed)
- 1/4 cup canned chickpeas (rinsed)
- 1 tbsp lemon juice
- Salt and pepper to taste

DIRECTIONS

1. Spread mashed avocado on the tortilla.
2. Add chickpeas and sprinkle with lemon juice.
3. Season with salt and pepper.
4. Roll up the tortilla into a wrap.
5. Serve immediately for a quick, filling lunch.

More Info :

Nutrition per Serving:
Calories: 290
Protein: 7g
Carbs: 40g
Fiber: 10g
Servings: 1
Cooking Time: 5 minutes

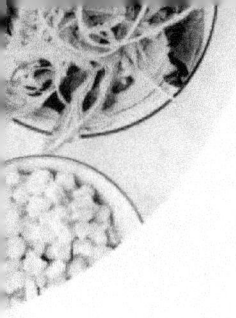

ROASTED VEGETABLE TACOS

INGREDIENTS

- 1/2 zucchini (sliced)
- 1/2 red bell pepper (sliced)
- 2 gluten-free corn tortillas
- 1 tbsp olive oil
- Salt and pepper to taste

DIRECTIONS

1. Preheat oven to 375°F (190°C).
2. Toss zucchini and bell pepper with olive oil, salt, and pepper.
3. Roast vegetables for 15 minutes until tender.
4. Warm tortillas and fill with roasted vegetables.
5. Serve with lime wedges for extra flavor.

More Info :

Nutrition per Serving:
Calories: 210
Protein: 5g
Carbs: 30g
Fiber: 5g
Servings: 1-2
Cooking Time: 20 minutes

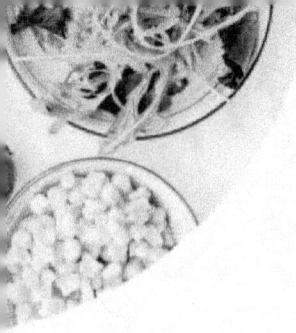

QUINOA AND ROASTED VEGGIE BOWL

INGREDIENTS

- 1/2 cup quinoa (cooked)
- 1/4 cup zucchini (sliced)
- 1/4 cup eggplant (diced)
- 1 tbsp olive oil
- 1 tbsp lemon juice
- Salt and pepper to taste

DIRECTIONS

1. Preheat oven to 375°F (190°C).
2. Toss zucchini and eggplant with olive oil, salt, and pepper.
3. Roast for 15 minutes until tender.
4. Mix roasted veggies with cooked quinoa.
5. Drizzle with lemon juice and serve.

More Info :

Nutrition per Serving:
Calories: 280
Protein: 8g
Carbs: 45g
Fiber: 6g
Servings: 1-2
Cooking Time: 20 minutes

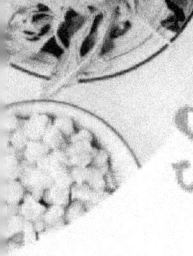

SPINACH AND FETA STUFFED PORTOBELLO MUSHROOMS

INGREDIENTS

- 2 large Portobello mushrooms (stems removed)
- 1/2 cup spinach (chopped)
- 2 tbsp feta cheese (crumbled)
- 1 tbsp olive oil
- Salt and pepper to taste

DIRECTIONS

1. Preheat oven to 350°F (175°C).
2. Sauté spinach in olive oil until wilted.
3. Stuff mushrooms with spinach and feta.
4. Bake for 15 minutes until mushrooms are tender.
5. Season with salt and pepper.
6. Serve hot.

More Info :

Nutrition per Serving:
Calories: 210
Protein: 6g
Carbs: 10g
Fiber: 4g
Servings: 1
Cooking Time: 20 minutes

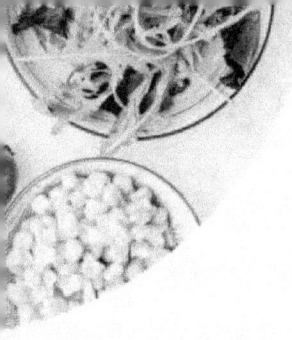

RICE NOODLE STIR-FRY

INGREDIENTS

- 1/2 cup rice noodles (cooked)
- 1/4 cup carrots (julienned)
- 1/4 cup bell peppers (sliced)
- 1 tbsp soy sauce (low sodium)
- 1 tbsp sesame oil

DIRECTIONS

1. Heat sesame oil in a pan over medium heat.
2. Add carrots and bell peppers, stir-fry for 3-4 minutes.
3. Toss in cooked rice noodles and soy sauce.
4. Stir-fry for another 2 minutes until well combined.
5. Serve hot and enjoy.
6. Optionally, top with sesame seeds.

More Info :

Nutrition per Serving:
Calories: 250
Protein: 4g
Carbs: 45g
Fiber: 3g
Servings: 1
Cooking Time: 10 minutes

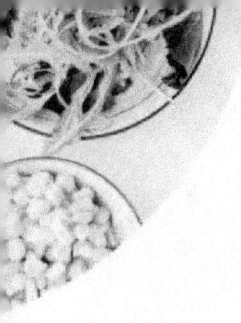

STUFFED ZUCCHINI BOATS

INGREDIENTS

- 1 zucchini (halved and scooped out)
- 1/2 cup quinoa (cooked)
- 1/4 cup tomatoes (diced)
- 1 tbsp olive oil
- Salt and pepper to taste

DIRECTIONS

1. Preheat oven to 375°F (190°C).
2. Mix cooked quinoa, tomatoes, and olive oil.
3. Stuff the zucchini halves with the quinoa mixture.
4. Bake for 15-20 minutes until tender.
5. Season with salt and pepper.
6. Serve hot.

More Info :

Nutrition per Serving:
Calories: 230
Protein: 6g
Carbs: 35g
Fiber: 5g
Servings: 1-2
Cooking Time: 20 minutes

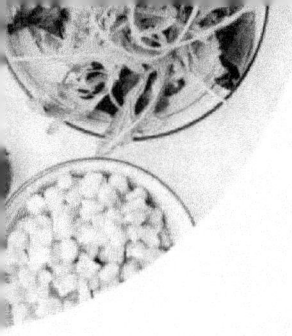

EGGPLANT AND LENTIL STEW

INGREDIENTS

- 1/2 eggplant (diced)
- 1/2 cup canned lentils (rinsed)
- 1 cup vegetable broth (low-FODMAP)
- 1 tbsp olive oil
- Salt and pepper to taste

DIRECTIONS

1. Heat olive oil in a pot over medium heat.
2. Add diced eggplant and sauté until soft.
3. Stir in lentils and vegetable broth.
4. Simmer for 15 minutes until stew thickens.
5. Season with salt and pepper.
6. Serve warm.

More Info :

Nutrition per Serving:
Calories: 210
Protein: 8g
Carbs: 35g
Fiber: 9g
Servings: 1-2
Cooking Time: 20 minutes

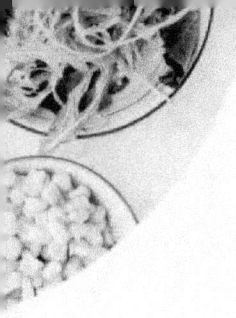

SWEET POTATO AND CHICKPEA SALAD

INGREDIENTS

- 1 medium sweet potato (diced)
- 1/2 cup canned chickpeas (rinsed)
- 1 tbsp olive oil
- 1 tbsp lemon juice
- Salt and pepper to taste

DIRECTIONS

1. Preheat oven to 375°F (190°C).
2. Toss sweet potatoes with olive oil, salt, and pepper, and roast for 20 minutes.
3. Mix roasted sweet potato and chickpeas in a bowl.
4. Drizzle with lemon juice and toss.
5. Serve warm or chilled.

More Info :

Nutrition per Serving:
Calories: 280
Protein: 8g
Carbs: 45g
Fiber: 10g
Servings: 1
Cooking Time: 25 minutes

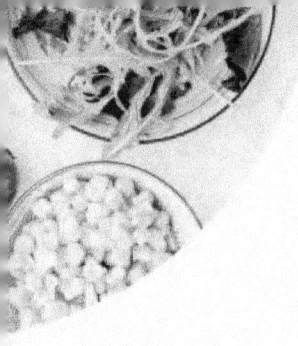

GRILLED TOFU WITH VEGGIES

INGREDIENTS

- 1/2 block firm tofu (cubed)
- 1/4 cup zucchini (sliced)
- 1/4 cup bell peppers (sliced)
- 1 tbsp soy sauce (low sodium)
- 1 tbsp olive oil

DIRECTIONS

1. Heat olive oil in a grill pan over medium heat.
2. Grill tofu cubes until golden brown.
3. Add zucchini and bell peppers, grill for 5-6 minutes.
4. Drizzle with soy sauce and toss.
5. Serve hot with additional veggies on the side.

More Info :

Nutrition per Serving:
Calories: 250
Protein: 12g
Carbs: 12g
Fiber: 4g
Servings: 1
Cooking Time: 15 minutes

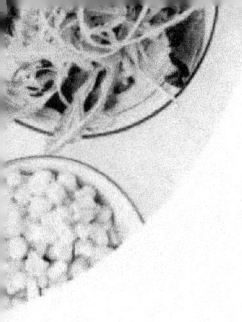

VEGETARIAN TACO SALAD

INGREDIENTS

- 1 cup romaine lettuce (chopped)
- 1/4 cup canned lentils (rinsed)
- 1/4 cup tomatoes (diced)
- 1 tbsp olive oil
- 1 tbsp lime juice

DIRECTIONS

1. In a bowl, combine lettuce, lentils, and tomatoes.
2. Drizzle with olive oil and lime juice.
3. Toss gently to combine.
4. Season with salt and pepper to taste.
5. Serve immediately for a light, refreshing lunch.

More Info :

Nutrition per Serving:
Calories: 180
Protein: 7g
Carbs: 20g
Fiber: 6g
Servings: 1
Cooking Time: 5 minutes

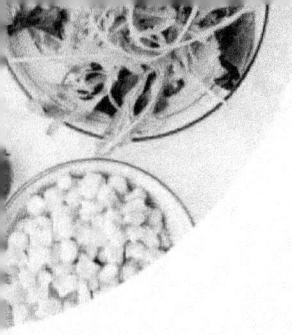

TOMATO AND AVOCADO WRAP

INGREDIENTS

- 1 gluten-free tortilla
- 1/2 avocado (sliced)
- 1/4 cup tomatoes (diced)
- 1 tbsp lemon juice
- Salt and pepper to taste

DIRECTIONS

1. Spread avocado slices on the tortilla.
2. Add diced tomatoes and sprinkle with lemon juice.
3. Season with salt and pepper.
4. Roll up the tortilla into a wrap.
5. Serve immediately for a quick, satisfying lunch.

More Info :

Nutrition per Serving:
Calories: 240
Protein: 4g
Carbs: 35g
Fiber: 8g
Servings: 1
Cooking Time: 5 minutes

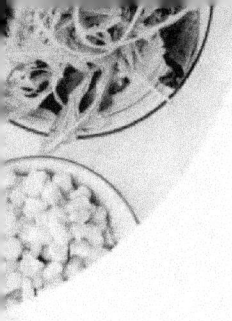

COCONUT CURRY
VEGETABLES

INGREDIENTS

- 1/2 cup carrots (sliced)
- 1/2 cup zucchini (sliced)
- 1/2 cup coconut milk (unsweetened)
- 1 tsp curry powder
- Salt and pepper to taste

DIRECTIONS

1. Heat coconut milk in a pot over medium heat.
2. Stir in curry powder and simmer for 2 minutes.
3. Add carrots and zucchini, cook for 10 minutes until tender.
4. Season with salt and pepper to taste.
5. Serve hot over rice or quinoa if desired.

More Info :

Nutrition per Serving:
Calories: 200
Protein: 3g
Carbs: 18g
Fiber: 5g
Servings: 1
Cooking Time: 15 minutes

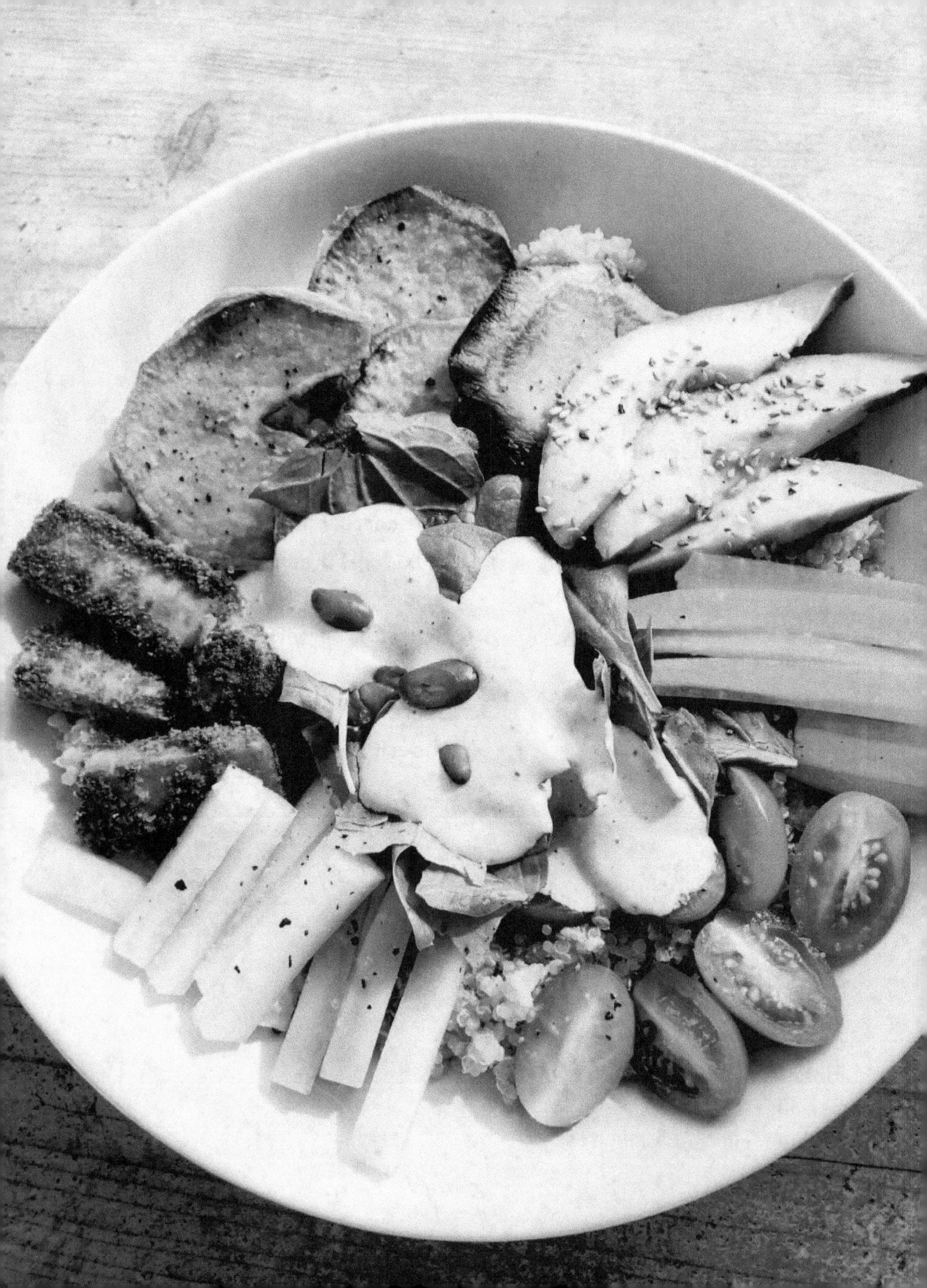

Dinner

Recipes

HERE ARE SIMPLE, LOW FODMAP DINNER
RECIPES, EACH WITH ITS INGREDIENTS,
DIRECTIONS, NUTRITIONAL INFORMATION,
SERVINGS, AND COOKING TIME.

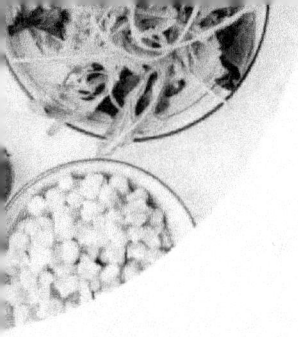

VEGETARIAN STIR-FRY WITH TOFU

INGREDIENTS

- 1/2 block firm tofu (cubed)
- 1/2 cup carrots (sliced)
- 1/2 cup zucchini (sliced)
- 1 tbsp olive oil
- 1 tbsp soy sauce (low sodium)
- 1 tbsp sesame seeds

DIRECTIONS

1. Heat olive oil in a pan over medium heat.
2. Stir-fry tofu until golden brown.
3. Add carrots and zucchini, cooking for 5-6 minutes.
4. Drizzle with soy sauce and toss.
5. Sprinkle with sesame seeds before serving.
6. Serve hot with rice or quinoa.

More Info :

Nutrition per Serving:
Calories: 240
Protein: 12g
Carbs: 18g
Fiber: 5g
Servings: 1
Cooking Time: 15 minutes

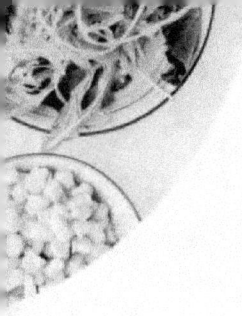

VEGETABLE LENTIL CURRY

INGREDIENTS

- 1/2 cup canned lentils (rinsed)
- 1/4 cup carrots (diced)
- 1/4 cup spinach (chopped)
- 1 cup coconut milk (unsweetened)
- 1 tbsp curry powder

DIRECTIONS

1. Heat coconut milk in a pot over medium heat.
2. Stir in curry powder and bring to a simmer.
3. Add lentils, carrots, and spinach, cooking for 10 minutes.
4. Stir occasionally until vegetables are tender.
5. Season with salt and pepper to taste.
6. Serve warm with rice or quinoa.

More Info :

Nutrition per Serving:
Calories: 280
Protein: 10g
Carbs: 40g
Fiber: 8g
Servings: 2
Cooking Time: 20 minutes

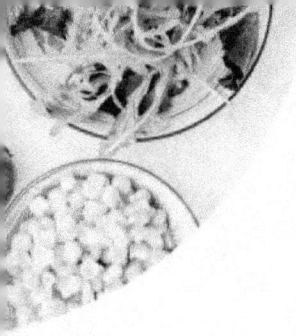

STUFFED BELL PEPPERS WITH QUINOA

INGREDIENTS

- 2 large bell peppers (halved and cored)
- 1/2 cup cooked quinoa
- 1/4 cup canned lentils (rinsed)
- 1 tbsp olive oil
- Salt and pepper to taste

DIRECTIONS

1. Preheat oven to 350°F (175°C).
2. Mix quinoa, lentils, and olive oil in a bowl.
3. Stuff bell pepper halves with the quinoa mixture.
4. Bake for 20 minutes until peppers are tender.
5. Season with salt and pepper.
6. Serve warm.

More Info :

Nutrition per Serving:
Calories: 230
Protein: 9g
Carbs: 35g
Fiber: 6g
Servings: 2
Cooking Time: 25 minutes

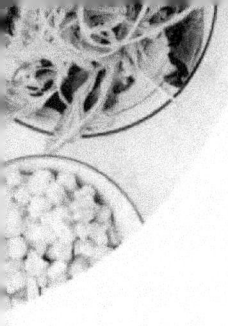

EGGPLANT STIR-FRY

INGREDIENTS

- 1/2 eggplant (diced)
- 1/2 cup red bell pepper (sliced)
- 1 tbsp olive oil
- 1 tbsp soy sauce (low sodium)
- Salt and pepper to taste

DIRECTIONS

1. Heat olive oil in a pan over medium heat.
2. Add eggplant and bell pepper, stir-fry for 5-6 minutes.
3. Drizzle with soy sauce and toss well.
4. Cook until vegetables are tender.
5. Season with salt and pepper to taste.
6. Serve hot with rice.

More Info :

Nutrition per Serving:
Calories: 180
Protein: 4g
Carbs: 20g
Fiber: 7g
Servings: 1
Cooking Time: 15 minutes

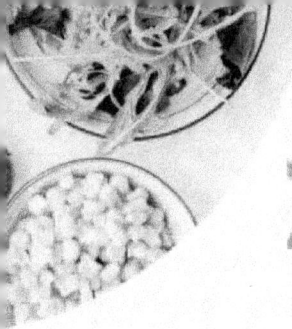

ZUCCHINI AND MUSHROOM RISOTTO

INGREDIENTS

- 1/2 cup Arborio rice
- 1/2 cup zucchini (sliced)
- 1/4 cup mushrooms (sliced)
- 1 1/2 cups vegetable broth (low-FODMAP)
- 1 tbsp olive oil

DIRECTIONS

1. Heat olive oil in a pan over medium heat.
2. Add rice and stir for 1-2 minutes.
3. Gradually add vegetable broth, stirring until absorbed.
4. Stir in zucchini and mushrooms, cook until rice is tender.
5. Season with salt and pepper.
6. Serve warm.

More Info :

Nutrition per Serving:
Calories: 280
Protein: 6g
Carbs: 50g
Fiber: 4g
Servings: 2
Cooking Time: 25 minutes

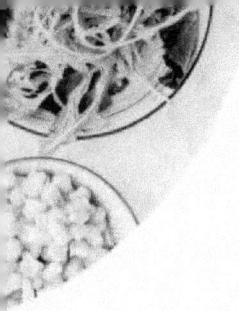

CHICKPEA AND SPINACH STEW

INGREDIENTS

- 1/2 cup canned chickpeas (rinsed)
- 1 cup spinach (chopped)
- 1 cup vegetable broth (low-FODMAP)
- 1 tbsp olive oil
- Salt and pepper to taste

DIRECTIONS

1. Heat olive oil in a pot over medium heat.
2. Add chickpeas and sauté for 3 minutes.
3. Pour in vegetable broth and bring to a simmer.
4. Add spinach and cook until wilted.
5. Season with salt and pepper to taste.
6. Serve hot.

More Info :

Nutrition per Serving:
Calories: 220
Protein: 9g
Carbs: 35g
Fiber: 7g
Servings: 1-2
Cooking Time: 15 minutes

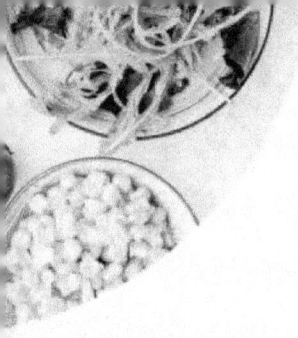

QUINOA AND ROASTED VEGETABLE BOWL

INGREDIENTS

- 1/2 cup quinoa (cooked)
- 1/2 zucchini (sliced)
- 1/2 cup bell peppers (sliced)
- 1 tbsp olive oil
- Salt and pepper to taste

DIRECTIONS

1. Preheat oven to 375°F (190°C).
2. Toss zucchini and bell peppers with olive oil, salt, and pepper.
3. Roast for 15 minutes until tender.
4. Mix roasted vegetables with cooked quinoa.
5. Serve warm and enjoy.

More Info :

Nutrition per Serving:
Calories: 260
Protein: 7g
Carbs: 45g
Fiber: 6g
Servings: 1-2
Cooking Time: 20 minutes

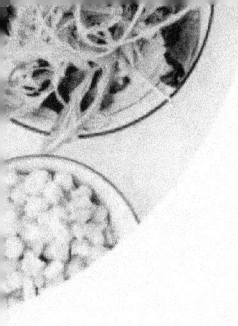

SWEET POTATO AND LENTIL SOUP

INGREDIENTS

- 1/2 cup sweet potato (diced)
- 1/2 cup canned lentils (rinsed)
- 2 cups vegetable broth (low-FODMAP)
- 1 tbsp olive oil
- Salt and pepper to taste

DIRECTIONS

1. Heat olive oil in a pot over medium heat.
2. Add diced sweet potato and cook for 5 minutes.
3. Pour in vegetable broth and bring to a simmer.
4. Add lentils and cook for 10 minutes until potatoes are tender.
5. Season with salt and pepper to taste.
6. Serve warm.

More Info :

Nutrition per Serving:
Calories: 250
Protein: 10g
Carbs: 45g
Fiber: 9g
Servings: 2
Cooking Time: 20 minutes

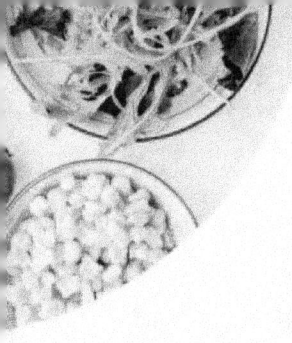

ROASTED VEGGIE TACOS

INGREDIENTS

- 1/2 zucchini (sliced)
- 1/4 cup carrots (sliced)
- 2 corn tortillas (gluten-free)
- 1 tbsp olive oil
- Salt and pepper to taste

DIRECTIONS

1. Preheat oven to 375°F (190°C).
2. Toss zucchini and carrots with olive oil, salt, and pepper.
3. Roast for 15 minutes until tender.
4. Warm tortillas and fill with roasted vegetables.
5. Serve with lime wedges if desired.

More Info :

Nutrition per Serving:
Calories: 200
Protein: 4g
Carbs: 30g
Fiber: 6g
Servings: 1
Cooking Time: 20 minutes

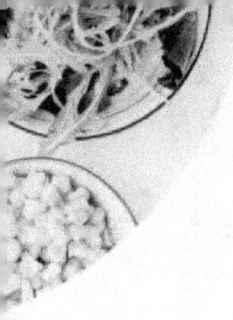

BAKED TOFU AND VEGETABLE SKEWERS

INGREDIENTS

- 1/2 block firm tofu (cubed)
- 1/4 cup bell peppers (sliced)
- 1/4 cup zucchini (sliced)
- 1 tbsp olive oil
- 1 tbsp soy sauce (low sodium)

DIRECTIONS

1. Preheat oven to 375°F (190°C).
2. Thread tofu, bell peppers, and zucchini onto skewers.
3. Drizzle with olive oil and soy sauce.
4. Bake for 15 minutes until vegetables are tender.
5. Serve with rice or quinoa.

More Info :

Nutrition per Serving:
Calories: 230
Protein: 11g
Carbs: 15g
Fiber: 4g
Servings: 1
Cooking Time: 20 minutes

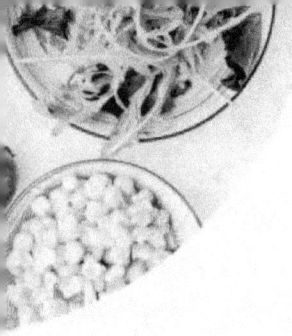

ROASTED SWEET POTATO AND QUINOA BOWL

INGREDIENTS

- 1 medium sweet potato (diced)
- 1/2 cup cooked quinoa
- 1/4 cup spinach (chopped)
- 1 tbsp olive oil
- 1 tbsp lemon juice
- Salt and pepper to taste

DIRECTIONS

1. Preheat oven to 375°F (190°C).
2. Toss diced sweet potatoes with olive oil, salt, and pepper.
3. Roast for 20 minutes until tender.
4. Combine roasted sweet potatoes, cooked quinoa, and spinach in a bowl.
5. Drizzle with lemon juice and toss.
6. Serve warm.

More Info :

Nutrition per Serving:
Calories: 300
Protein: 8g
Carbs: 50g
Fiber: 7g
Servings: 1-2
Cooking Time: 25 minutes

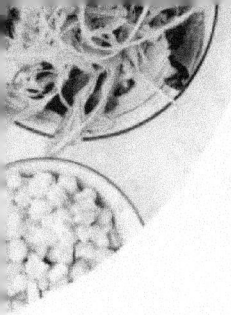

VEGETABLE AND CHICKPEA STIR-FRY

INGREDIENTS

- 1/2 cup canned chickpeas (rinsed)
- 1/2 cup carrots (sliced)
- 1/2 cup zucchini (sliced)
- 1 tbsp olive oil
- 1 tbsp soy sauce (low sodium)

DIRECTIONS

1. Heat olive oil in a pan over medium heat.
2. Add chickpeas, carrots, and zucchini; stir-fry for 5-6 minutes.
3. Drizzle with soy sauce and toss.
4. Cook until vegetables are tender.
5. Serve hot with rice or quinoa.

More Info :

Nutrition per Serving:
Calories: 280
Protein: 10g
Carbs: 40g
Fiber: 8g
Servings: 1
Cooking Time: 15 minutes

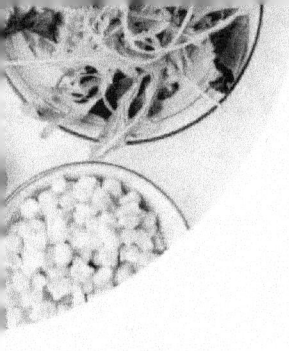

BAKED EGGPLANT PARMESAN

INGREDIENTS

- 1 small eggplant (sliced)
- 1/4 cup gluten-free breadcrumbs
- 2 tbsp Parmesan cheese (grated)
- 1 tbsp olive oil
- Salt and pepper to taste

DIRECTIONS

1. Preheat oven to 375°F (190°C).
2. Brush eggplant slices with olive oil and season with salt and pepper.
3. Coat eggplant in breadcrumbs and Parmesan cheese.
4. Bake for 20 minutes until crispy.
5. Serve with marinara sauce or as a side dish.

More Info :

Nutrition per Serving:
Calories: 220
Protein: 7g
Carbs: 30g
Fiber: 5g
Servings: 1-2
Cooking Time: 25 minutes

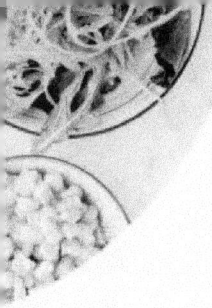

TOFU AND VEGETABLE KEBABS

INGREDIENTS

- 1/2 block firm tofu (cubed)
- 1/4 cup zucchini (sliced)
- 1/4 cup bell peppers (sliced)
- 1 tbsp olive oil
- 1 tbsp soy sauce (low sodium)

DIRECTIONS

1. Preheat oven to 375°F (190°C).
2. Thread tofu, zucchini, and bell peppers onto skewers.
3. Drizzle with olive oil and soy sauce.
4. Bake for 15 minutes until tender.
5. Serve with rice or salad.

More Info :

Nutrition per Serving:
Calories: 240
Protein: 10g
Carbs: 15g
Fiber: 5g
Servings: 1
Cooking Time: 20 minutes

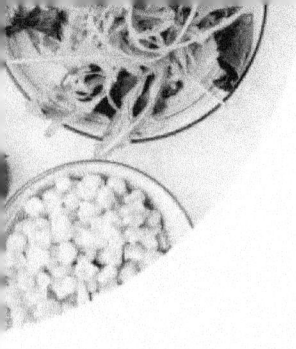

LENTIL AND SPINACH PASTA

INGREDIENTS

- 1/2 cup gluten-free pasta
- 1/4 cup canned lentils (rinsed)
- 1/2 cup spinach (chopped)
- 1 tbsp olive oil
- Salt and pepper to taste

DIRECTIONS

1. Cook pasta according to package instructions.
2. In a pan, sauté lentils and spinach in olive oil for 3-4 minutes.
3. Drain pasta and toss with the lentil-spinach mixture.
4. Season with salt and pepper to taste.
5. Serve hot and enjoy!
6. Optionally, sprinkle with Parmesan cheese.

More Info :

Nutrition per Serving:
Calories: 280
Protein: 10g
Carbs: 40g
Fiber: 8g
Servings: 1
Cooking Time: 15 minutes

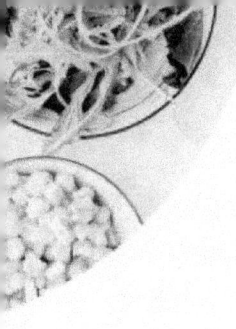

GRILLED ZUCCHINI AND CHICKPEA SALAD

INGREDIENTS

- 1/2 zucchini (sliced)
- 1/2 cup canned chickpeas (rinsed)
- 1 tbsp olive oil
- 1 tbsp lemon juice
- Salt and pepper to taste

DIRECTIONS

1. Heat olive oil in a grill pan over medium heat.
2. Grill zucchini slices until tender and slightly charred.
3. In a bowl, mix grilled zucchini, chickpeas, and lemon juice.
4. Season with salt and pepper.
5. Serve warm or chilled.

More Info :

Nutrition per Serving:
Calories: 250
Protein: 8g
Carbs: 35g
Fiber: 7g
Servings: 1
Cooking Time: 10 minutes

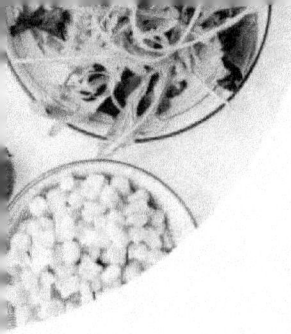

BAKED SWEET POTATO FRIES

INGREDIENTS

- 1 medium sweet potato (sliced into fries)
- 1 tbsp olive oil
- 1/2 tsp paprika
- Salt and pepper to taste

DIRECTIONS

1. Preheat oven to 400°F (200°C).
2. Toss sweet potato slices with olive oil, paprika, salt, and pepper.
3. Spread on a baking sheet and bake for 20 minutes until crispy.
4. Flip halfway through for even cooking.
5. Serve with your favorite dipping sauce.

More Info :

Nutrition per Serving:
Calories: 200
Protein: 3g
Carbs: 35g
Fiber: 6g
Servings: 1
Cooking Time: 25 minutes

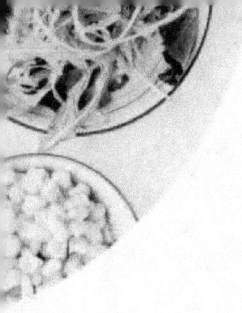

VEGETABLE AND TOFU SKILLET

INGREDIENTS

- 1/2 block firm tofu (cubed)
- 1/2 cup bell peppers (sliced)
- 1/2 cup zucchini (sliced)
- 1 tbsp olive oil
- Salt and pepper to taste

DIRECTIONS

1. Heat olive oil in a skillet over medium heat.
2. Cook tofu cubes until golden brown.
3. Add bell peppers and zucchini, sauté for 5-6 minutes.
4. Season with salt and pepper.
5. Serve hot with rice or quinoa.

More Info :

Nutrition per Serving:
Calories: 240
Protein: 12g
Carbs: 15g
Fiber: 4g
Servings: 1
Cooking Time: 15 minutes

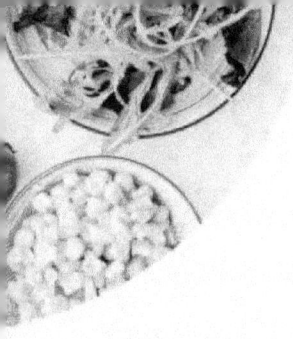

ROASTED CARROT AND LENTIL SALAD

INGREDIENTS

- 1/2 cup carrots (sliced)
- 1/2 cup canned lentils (rinsed)
- 1 tbsp olive oil
- 1 tbsp lemon juice
- Salt and pepper to taste

DIRECTIONS

1. Preheat oven to 375°F (190°C).
2. Toss carrot slices with olive oil, salt, and pepper.
3. Roast for 15 minutes until tender.
4. In a bowl, combine roasted carrots and lentils.
5. Drizzle with lemon juice and toss.
6. Serve warm or chilled.

More Info :

Nutrition per Serving:
Calories: 230
Protein: 8g
Carbs: 40g
Fiber: 9g
Servings: 1
Cooking Time: 20 minutes

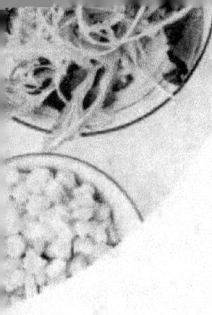

MUSHROOM AND SPINACH STIR-FRY

INGREDIENTS

- 1/2 cup mushrooms (sliced)
- 1/2 cup spinach (chopped)
- 1 tbsp olive oil
- 1 tbsp soy sauce (low sodium)
- Salt and pepper to taste

DIRECTIONS

1. Heat olive oil in a pan over medium heat.
2. Sauté mushrooms until golden brown, about 3-4 minutes.
3. Add spinach and cook until wilted.
4. Drizzle with soy sauce and toss well.
5. Season with salt and pepper to taste.
6. Serve hot with rice or quinoa.

More Info :

Nutrition per Serving:
Calories: 180
Protein: 6g
Carbs: 20g
Fiber: 4g
Servings: 1
Cooking Time: 10 minutes

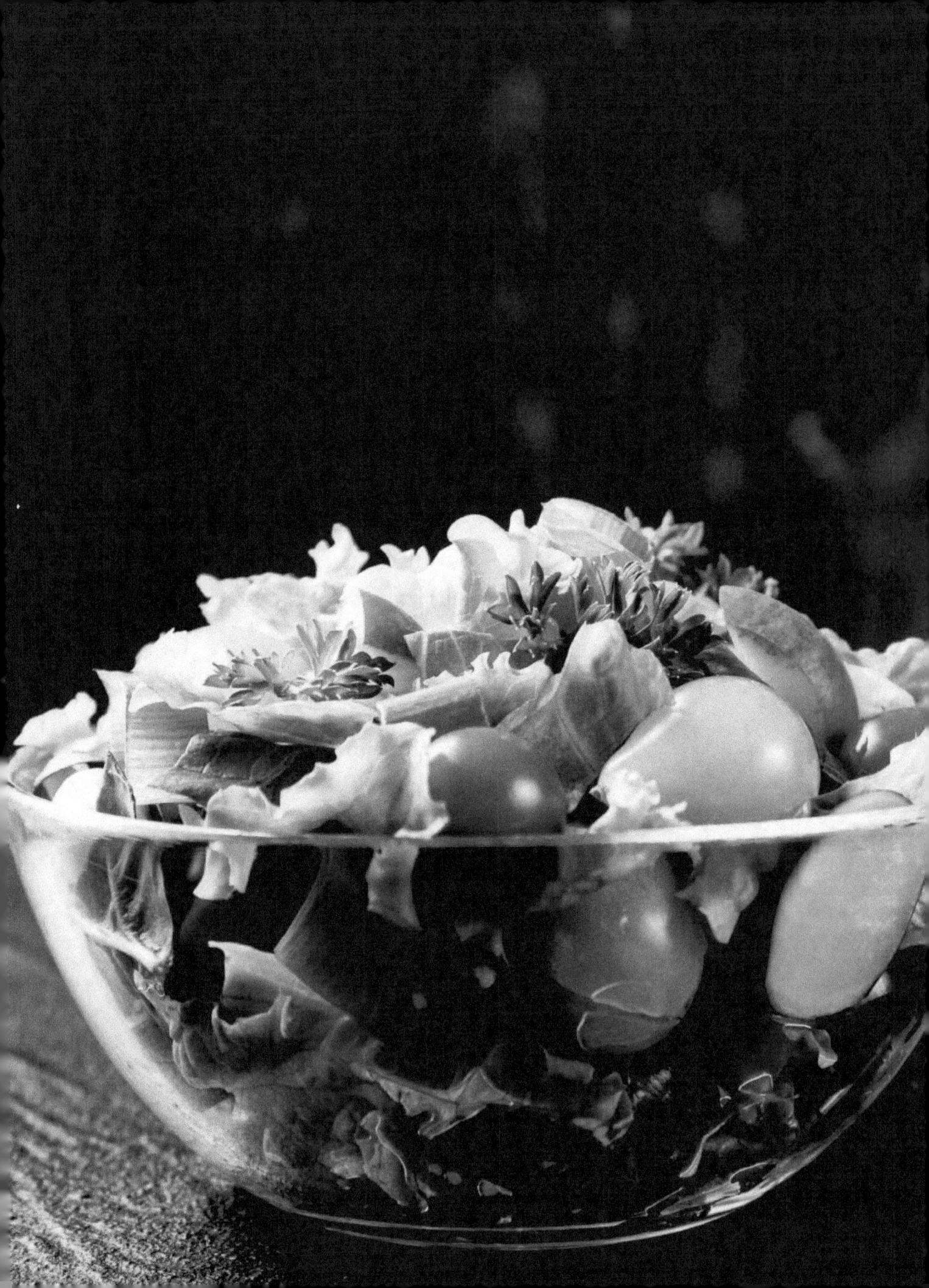

Snacks Recipes

HERE ARE SIMPLE, LOW FODMAP SNACKS RECIPES, EACH WITH ITS INGREDIENTS, DIRECTIONS, NUTRITIONAL INFORMATION, SERVINGS, AND COOKING TIME.

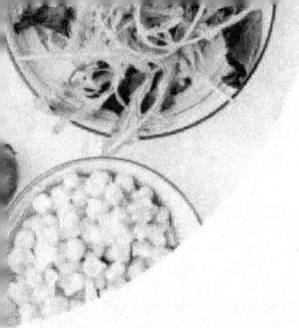

CUCUMBER AND AVOCADO BITES

INGREDIENTS

- 1 cucumber (sliced)
- 1/2 avocado (mashed)
- 1 tbsp lemon juice
- Salt and pepper to taste

DIRECTIONS

1. Slice the cucumber into rounds.
2. Mash avocado and mix with lemon juice.
3. Spread the avocado mixture on top of each cucumber slice.
4. Sprinkle with salt and pepper.
5. Serve immediately as a refreshing snack.

More Info :

Nutrition per Serving:
Calories: 100
Protein: 2g
Carbs: 10g
Fiber: 4g
Servings: 1-2
Cooking Time: 5 minutes

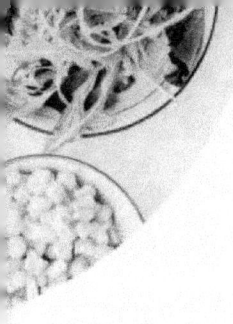

ZUCCHINI CHIPS

INGREDIENTS

- 1 medium zucchini (sliced thinly)
- 1 tbsp olive oil
- 1/2 tsp paprika
- Salt and pepper to taste

DIRECTIONS

1. Preheat oven to 375°F (190°C).
2. Toss zucchini slices with olive oil, paprika, salt, and pepper.
3. Arrange slices on a baking sheet in a single layer.
4. Bake for 15-20 minutes until crispy.
5. Allow to cool slightly before serving.
6. Enjoy as a crunchy, healthy snack.

More Info :

Nutrition per Serving:
Calories: 90
Protein: 2g
Carbs: 10g
Fiber: 2g
Servings: 1
Cooking Time: 20 minutes

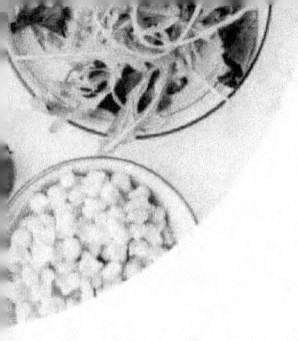

CARROT STICKS WITH PEANUT BUTTER

INGREDIENTS

- 2 medium carrots (cut into sticks)
- 2 tbsp peanut butter (unsweetened)
- 1 tbsp chia seeds

DIRECTIONS

1. Cut carrots into sticks.
2. Serve peanut butter in a small bowl.
3. Sprinkle chia seeds over the peanut butter.
4. Dip carrot sticks into peanut butter for a nutritious snack.
5. Enjoy immediately.

More Info :

Nutrition per Serving:
Calories: 220
Protein: 7g
Carbs: 18g
Fiber: 6g
Servings: 1
Cooking Time: 5 minutes

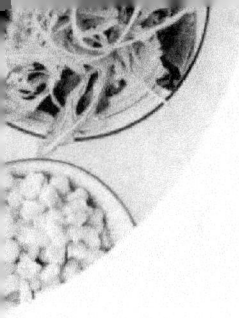

BANANA OAT ENERGY BITES

INGREDIENTS

- 1 ripe banana (mashed)
- 1 cup gluten-free rolled oats
- 1 tbsp chia seeds
- 1 tbsp maple syrup

DIRECTIONS

1. Mash the banana in a bowl.
2. Add oats, chia seeds, and maple syrup.
3. Mix well and form into small balls.
4. Place in the fridge to chill for 30 minutes.
5. Enjoy as an energy-boosting snack.
6. Keep refrigerated for freshness.

More Info :

Nutrition per Serving:
Calories: 160
Protein: 4g
Carbs: 30g
Fiber: 5g
Servings: 2
Cooking Time: 5 minutes (plus chilling)

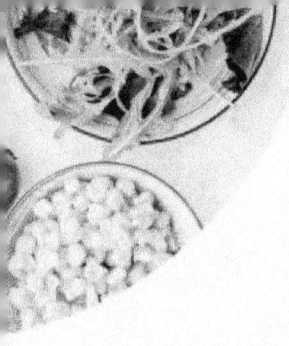

COCONUT CHIA PUDDING

INGREDIENTS

- 2 tbsp chia seeds
- 1/2 cup coconut milk (unsweetened)
- 1 tsp maple syrup
- 1/4 cup blueberries

DIRECTIONS

1. In a bowl, mix chia seeds, coconut milk, and maple syrup.
2. Stir well to avoid clumps.
3. Refrigerate for at least 4 hours or overnight.
4. Top with blueberries before serving.
5. Enjoy chilled as a creamy snack.

More Info :

Nutrition per Serving:
Calories: 180
Protein: 4g
Carbs: 15g
Fiber: 8g
Servings: 1
Cooking Time: 5 minutes (plus chilling)

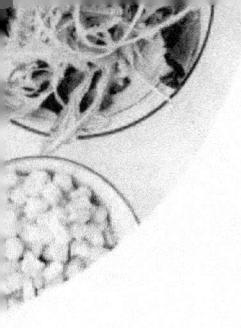

RICE CAKES WITH ALMOND BUTTER

INGREDIENTS

- 2 plain rice cakes
- 2 tbsp almond butter
- 1 tbsp chia seeds

DIRECTIONS

1. Spread almond butter evenly over the rice cakes.
2. Sprinkle chia seeds on top.
3. Serve immediately as a quick snack.
4. Enjoy the combination of crunchy and creamy textures.
5. Ideal for a quick energy boost.

More Info :

Nutrition per Serving:
Calories: 200
Protein: 6g
Carbs: 24g
Fiber: 5g
Servings: 1
Cooking Time: 3 minutes

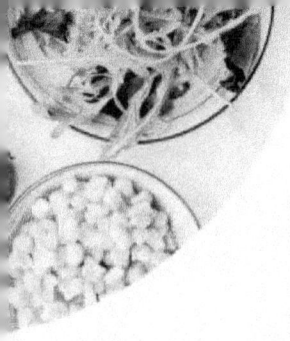

BAKED KALE
CHIPS

INGREDIENTS

- 1 cup kale (stems removed and leaves torn)
- 1 tbsp olive oil
- 1/2 tsp sea salt

DIRECTIONS

1. Preheat oven to 350°F (175°C).
2. Toss kale with olive oil and sea salt.
3. Spread kale leaves on a baking sheet.
4. Bake for 10-15 minutes until crispy.
5. Allow to cool before serving.

More Info :

Nutrition per Serving:
Calories: 90
Protein: 3g
Carbs: 7g
Fiber: 2g
Servings: 1
Cooking Time: 15 minutes

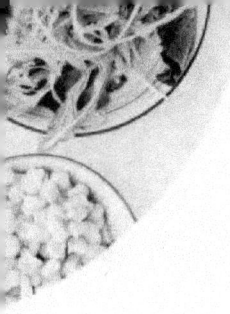

ROASTED CHICKPEAS

INGREDIENTS

- 1/2 cup canned chickpeas (rinsed)
- 1 tbsp olive oil
- 1/2 tsp paprika
- Salt and pepper to taste

DIRECTIONS

1. Preheat oven to 400°F (200°C).
2. Toss chickpeas with olive oil, paprika, salt, and pepper.
3. Spread on a baking sheet and roast for 20-25 minutes.
4. Stir halfway through to ensure even cooking.
5. Let cool before serving.

More Info :

Nutrition per Serving:
Calories: 200
Protein: 7g
Carbs: 25g
Fiber: 8g
Servings: 1
Cooking Time: 25 minutes

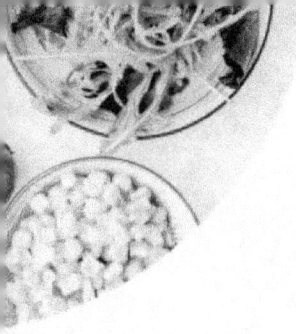

STUFFED MINI BELL PEPPERS

INGREDIENTS

- 6 mini bell peppers (halved and seeded)
- 1/4 cup lactose-free cream cheese
- 1 tbsp chives (chopped)
- Salt and pepper to taste

DIRECTIONS

1. Cut mini bell peppers in half and remove seeds.
2. In a bowl, mix cream cheese and chives.
3. Spoon the mixture into each bell pepper half.
4. Season with salt and pepper.
5. Serve immediately as a crunchy, creamy snack.

More Info :

Nutrition per Serving:
Calories: 120
Protein: 4g
Carbs: 10g
Fiber: 3g
Servings: 2
Cooking Time: 5 minutes

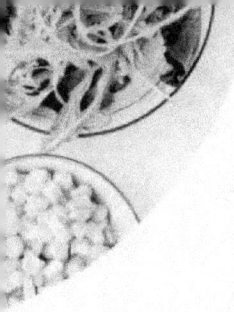

APPLE SLICES WITH SUNFLOWER SEED BUTTER

INGREDIENTS

- 1 apple (sliced)
- 2 tbsp sunflower seed butter
- 1 tsp chia seeds

DIRECTIONS

1. Slice the apple into rounds or wedges.
2. Spread sunflower seed butter on each apple slice.
3. Sprinkle chia seeds on top for added crunch.
4. Serve immediately.

More Info :

Nutrition per Serving:
Calories: 220
Protein: 4g
Carbs: 30g
Fiber: 6g
Servings: 1
Cooking Time: 5 minutes

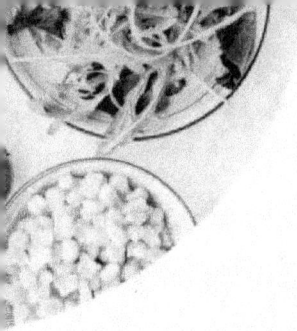

PEANUT BUTTER BANANA BITES

INGREDIENTS

- 1 banana (sliced)
- 2 tbsp peanut butter (unsweetened)
- 1 tbsp chia seeds

DIRECTIONS

1. Slice the banana into rounds.
2. Spread a small amount of peanut butter on each slice.
3. Sprinkle chia seeds over the peanut butter.
4. Stack banana slices to make mini sandwiches if desired.
5. Serve immediately for a quick, protein-packed snack.

More Info :

Nutrition per Serving:
Calories: 220
Protein: 6g
Carbs: 28g
Fiber: 5g
Servings: 1
Cooking Time: 5 minutes

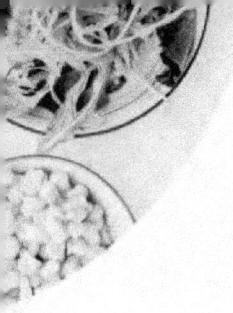

CRISPY BAKED TOFU CUBES

INGREDIENTS

- 1/2 block firm tofu (cubed)
- 1 tbsp olive oil
- 1/2 tsp paprika
- Salt and pepper to taste

DIRECTIONS

1. Preheat oven to 375°F (190°C).
2. Toss tofu cubes with olive oil, paprika, salt, and pepper.
3. Spread cubes on a baking sheet.
4. Bake for 20 minutes, flipping halfway through.
5. Serve warm and enjoy as a protein-rich snack.
6. Optionally, serve with a low-FODMAP dipping sauce.

More Info :

Nutrition per Serving:
Calories: 180
Protein: 12g
Carbs: 5g
Fiber: 3g
Servings: 1
Cooking Time: 20 minutes

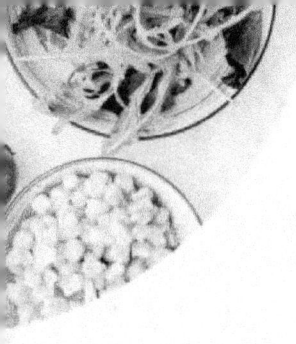

CUCUMBER ROLL-UPS WITH CREAM CHEESE

INGREDIENTS

- 1 cucumber (sliced thinly)
- 1/4 cup lactose-free cream cheese
- 1 tbsp chives (chopped)
- Salt and pepper to taste

DIRECTIONS

1. Slice the cucumber lengthwise into thin strips.
2. Spread cream cheese on each cucumber strip.
3. Sprinkle with chives and season with salt and pepper.
4. Roll up the cucumber strips and secure with a toothpick.
5. Serve chilled and enjoy as a refreshing snack.

More Info :

Nutrition per Serving:
Calories: 120
Protein: 4g
Carbs: 7g
Fiber: 2g
Servings: 1
Cooking Time: 5 minutes

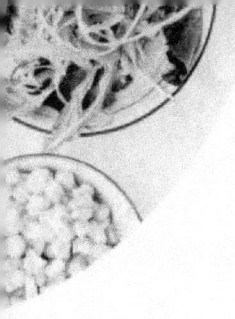

CHIA SEED CRACKERS

INGREDIENTS

- 1/2 cup chia seeds
- 1/2 cup water
- 1/2 tsp sea salt
- 1/2 tsp garlic-infused oil (optional)

DIRECTIONS

1. Preheat oven to 325°F (160°C).
2. Mix chia seeds, water, and sea salt in a bowl.
3. Let the mixture sit for 10 minutes until it forms a gel.
4. Spread the mixture thinly on a baking sheet.
5. Bake for 30 minutes until crispy.
6. Break into pieces and serve as crunchy crackers.

More Info :

Nutrition per Serving:
Calories: 180
Protein: 6g
Carbs: 12g
Fiber: 9g
Servings: 2
Cooking Time: 40 minutes

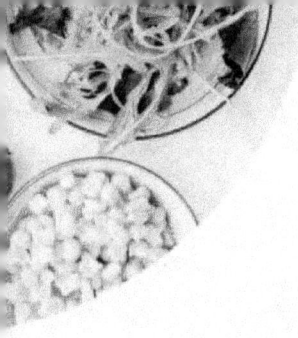

ROASTED PUMPKIN SEEDS

INGREDIENTS

- 1/2 cup pumpkin seeds
- 1 tbsp olive oil
- 1/2 tsp sea salt
- 1/2 tsp paprika

DIRECTIONS

1. Preheat oven to 350°F (175°C).
2. Toss pumpkin seeds with olive oil, sea salt, and paprika.
3. Spread seeds on a baking sheet in a single layer.
4. Bake for 15 minutes until golden and crispy.
5. Let cool slightly before serving.

More Info :

Nutrition per Serving:
Calories: 160
Protein: 8g
Carbs: 5g
Fiber: 4g
Servings: 1
Cooking Time: 15 minutes

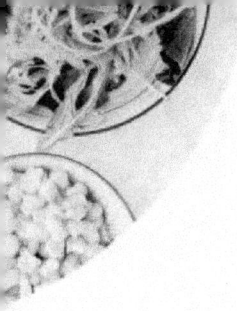

STRAWBERRY COCONUT BITES

INGREDIENTS

- 1/2 cup strawberries (sliced)
- 2 tbsp shredded coconut (unsweetened)
- 1 tbsp maple syrup

DIRECTIONS

1. Slice the strawberries into small pieces.
2. Roll strawberries in shredded coconut.
3. Drizzle with maple syrup.
4. Serve immediately as a naturally sweet snack.
5. Enjoy for a quick, healthy treat.

More Info :

Nutrition per Serving:
Calories: 100
Protein: 1g
Carbs: 20g
Fiber: 3g
Servings: 1
Cooking Time: 5 minutes

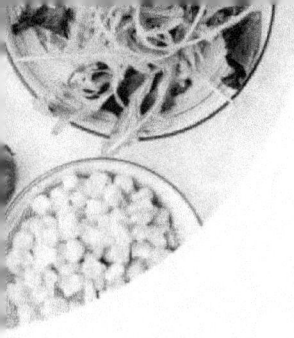

OATMEAL SNACK BARS

INGREDIENTS

- 1 cup gluten-free rolled oats
- 1/4 cup peanut butter (unsweetened)
- 2 tbsp maple syrup
- 1/4 cup chia seeds

DIRECTIONS

1. Preheat oven to 350°F (175°C).
2. Mix oats, peanut butter, maple syrup, and chia seeds in a bowl.
3. Press the mixture into a lined baking dish.
4. Bake for 15-20 minutes until firm.
5. Let cool and cut into bars.

More Info :

Nutrition per Serving:
Calories: 180
Protein: 6g
Carbs: 24g
Fiber: 6g
Servings: 2-3
Cooking Time: 20 minutes

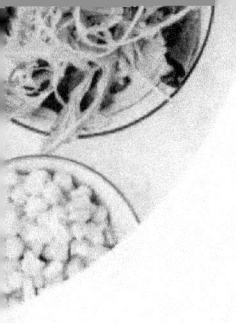

CRISPY ROASTED KALE

INGREDIENTS

- 1 cup kale (stems removed and leaves torn)
- 1 tbsp olive oil
- 1/2 tsp sea salt
- 1/2 tsp garlic-infused oil (optional)

DIRECTIONS

1. Preheat oven to 350°F (175°C).
2. Toss kale with olive oil and sea salt.
3. Spread kale leaves on a baking sheet.
4. Bake for 10-15 minutes until crispy.
5. Serve immediately for a light, crunchy snack.

More Info :

Nutrition per Serving:
Calories: 80
Protein: 3g
Carbs: 7g
Fiber: 2g
Servings: 1
Cooking Time: 15 minutes

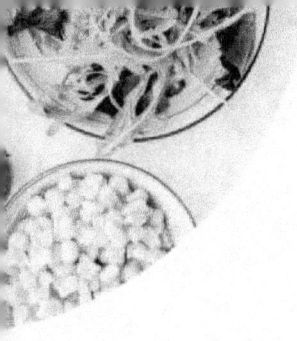

BLUEBERRY ALMOND PARFAIT

INGREDIENTS

- 1/2 cup lactose-free yogurt
- 1/4 cup blueberries
- 1 tbsp slivered almonds
- 1 tsp maple syrup

DIRECTIONS

1. Layer yogurt, blueberries, and almonds in a glass.
2. Drizzle with maple syrup for sweetness.
3. Serve immediately for a protein-packed snack.
4. Enjoy this light and refreshing parfait.

More Info :

Nutrition per Serving:
Calories: 150
Protein: 6g
Carbs: 18g
Fiber: 3g
Servings: 1
Cooking Time: 5 minutes

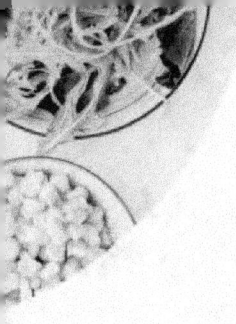

SESAME SEED CRACKERS

INGREDIENTS

- 1/4 cup sesame seeds
- 1/4 cup gluten-free flour
- 1 tbsp olive oil
- 1/2 tsp sea salt

DIRECTIONS

1. Preheat oven to 350°F (175°C).
2. Mix sesame seeds, gluten-free flour, olive oil, and sea salt.
3. Form the dough into small balls and flatten them onto a baking sheet.
4. Bake for 10-12 minutes until golden and crisp.
5. Let cool before serving as a crunchy snack.
6. Enjoy with your favorite dip.

More Info :

Nutrition per Serving:
Calories: 140
Protein: 4g
Carbs: 12g
Fiber: 4g
Servings: 1-2
Cooking Time: 12 minutes

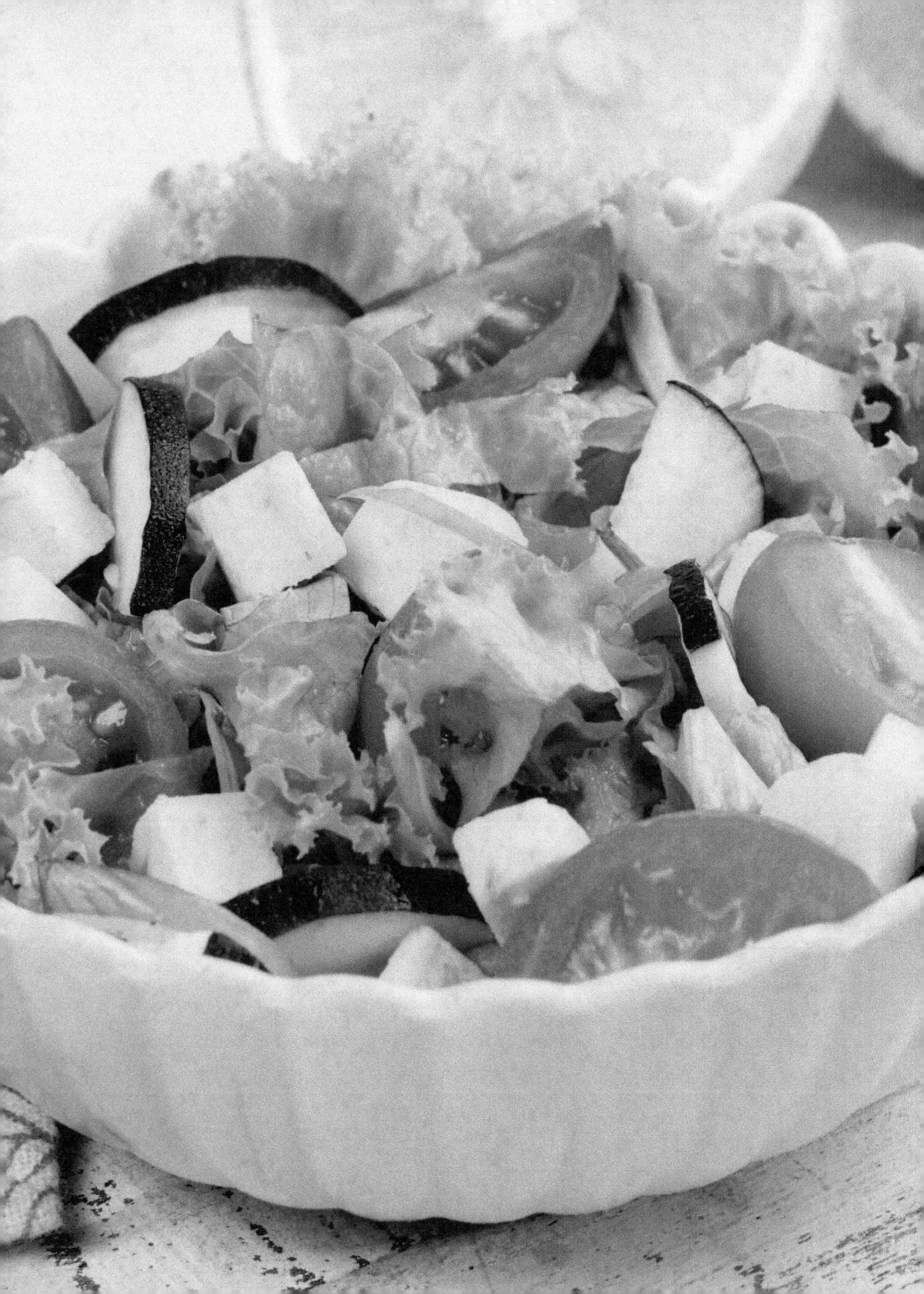

Dessert Recipes

HERE ARE SIMPLE, LOW FODMAP DESSERT RECIPES, EACH WITH ITS INGREDIENTS, DIRECTIONS, NUTRITIONAL INFORMATION, SERVINGS, AND COOKING TIME.

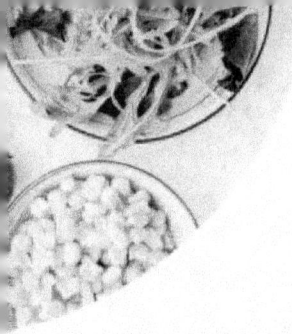

COCONUT
MACAROONS

INGREDIENTS

- 1 1/2 cups shredded coconut (unsweetened)
- 1/4 cup maple syrup
- 1 tsp vanilla extract
- 1 tbsp chia seeds

DIRECTIONS

1. Preheat oven to 350°F (175°C).
2. In a bowl, mix shredded coconut, maple syrup, vanilla, and chia seeds.
3. Form small balls and place on a lined baking sheet.
4. Bake for 12-15 minutes until golden.
5. Let cool before serving.

More Info :

Nutrition per Serving:
Calories: 200
Protein: 3g
Carbs: 20g
Fiber: 4g
Servings: 2-3
Cooking Time: 15 minutes

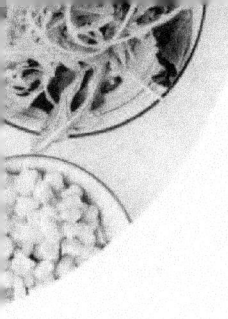

BANANA NICE CREAM

INGREDIENTS

- 2 ripe bananas (frozen)
- 1 tbsp almond butter
- 1/2 tsp vanilla extract

DIRECTIONS

1. Place frozen bananas in a blender or food processor.
2. Blend until smooth and creamy.
3. Add almond butter and vanilla extract, blend until combined.
4. Serve immediately as a healthy, dairy-free ice cream.
5. Enjoy this quick and easy treat.

More Info :

Nutrition per Serving:
Calories: 180
Protein: 2g
Carbs: 35g
Fiber: 5g
Servings: 1-2
Cooking Time: 5 minutes

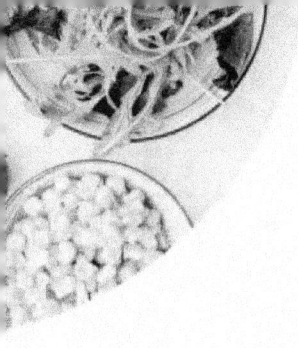

BLUEBERRY CHIA PUDDING

INGREDIENTS

- 1/4 cup chia seeds
- 1 cup almond milk (unsweetened)
- 1 tbsp maple syrup
- 1/4 cup blueberries

DIRECTIONS

1. Mix chia seeds, almond milk, and maple syrup in a bowl.
2. Stir well and refrigerate for 4 hours or overnight.
3. Stir again before serving.
4. Top with fresh blueberries.
5. Enjoy a creamy and nutritious dessert.

More Info :

Nutrition per Serving:
Calories: 160
Protein: 4g
Carbs: 22g
Fiber: 10g
Servings: 2
Cooking Time: 5 minutes (plus chilling)

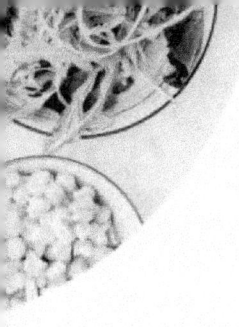

CHOCOLATE AVOCADO MOUSSE

INGREDIENTS

- 1 ripe avocado
- 2 tbsp cocoa powder (unsweetened)
- 2 tbsp maple syrup
- 1/2 tsp vanilla extract

DIRECTIONS

1. Blend avocado, cocoa powder, maple syrup, and vanilla until smooth.
2. Spoon into small bowls.
3. Refrigerate for 1 hour before serving.
4. Enjoy this rich and creamy mousse.

More Info :

Nutrition per Serving:
Calories: 230
Protein: 3g
Carbs: 24g
Fiber: 8g
Servings: 2
Cooking Time: 5 minutes (plus chilling)

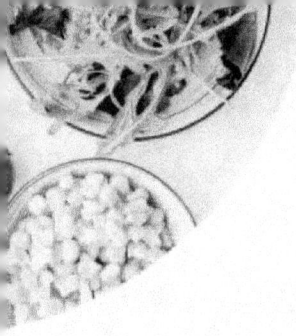

LACTOSE-FREE YOGURT PARFAIT

INGREDIENTS

- 1/2 cup lactose-free yogurt
- 1/4 cup strawberries (sliced)
- 1 tbsp chia seeds
- 1 tsp maple syrup

DIRECTIONS

1. Layer yogurt, strawberries, and chia seeds in a glass.
2. Drizzle with maple syrup.
3. Serve immediately as a light and healthy dessert.
4. Enjoy this refreshing parfait.

More Info :

Nutrition per Serving:
Calories: 150
Protein: 6g
Carbs: 20g
Fiber: 4g
Servings: 1
Cooking Time: 5 minutes

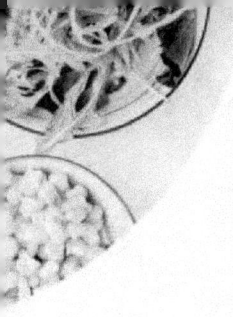

COCONUT RICE PUDDING

INGREDIENTS

- 1/2 cup jasmine rice (cooked)
- 1 cup coconut milk (unsweetened)
- 1 tbsp maple syrup
- 1/2 tsp cinnamon

DIRECTIONS

1. In a pot, combine cooked rice, coconut milk, and maple syrup.
2. Simmer for 10 minutes, stirring occasionally.
3. Stir in cinnamon and cook until thick and creamy.
4. Serve warm or chilled for a comforting dessert.

More Info :

Nutrition per Serving:
Calories: 220
Protein: 3g
Carbs: 35g
Fiber: 3g
Servings: 1-2
Cooking Time: 15 minutes

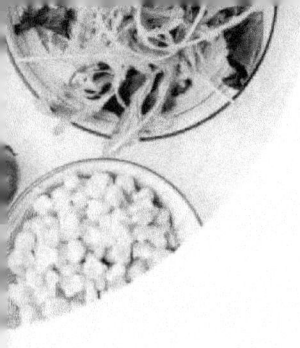

CHOCOLATE-DIPPED STRAWBERRIES

INGREDIENTS

- 1/2 cup dark chocolate (dairy-free)
- 1/2 cup strawberries (whole)

DIRECTIONS

1. Melt dark chocolate in a microwave-safe bowl.
2. Dip strawberries into the melted chocolate.
3. Place on a baking sheet lined with parchment paper.
4. Refrigerate until the chocolate hardens.
5. Serve chilled for a simple, indulgent treat.

More Info :

Nutrition per Serving:
Calories: 160
Protein: 2g
Carbs: 22g
Fiber: 5g
Servings: 2
Cooking Time: 10 minutes (plus chilling)

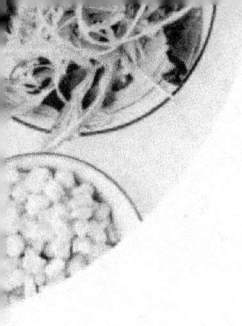

PEANUT BUTTER CHOCOLATE BITES

INGREDIENTS

- 1/4 cup peanut butter (unsweetened)
- 2 tbsp cocoa powder (unsweetened)
- 2 tbsp maple syrup
- 1 tbsp chia seeds

DIRECTIONS

1. Mix peanut butter, cocoa powder, maple syrup, and chia seeds in a bowl.
2. Roll the mixture into small balls.
3. Refrigerate for 30 minutes before serving.
4. Enjoy these chocolatey, no-bake bites.

More Info :

Nutrition per Serving:
Calories: 200
Protein: 5g
Carbs: 15g
Fiber: 5g
Servings: 2
Cooking Time: 5 minutes (plus chilling)

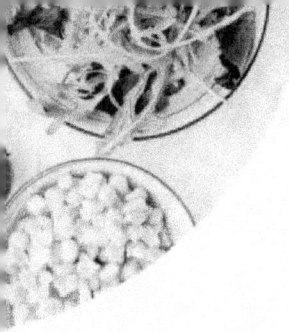

MANGO SORBET

INGREDIENTS

- 1 cup frozen mango chunks
- 1 tbsp lime juice
- 1 tbsp maple syrup

DIRECTIONS

1. Blend frozen mango chunks, lime juice, and maple syrup until smooth.
2. Spoon into bowls.
3. Serve immediately as a refreshing sorbet.
4. Enjoy this tropical treat.

More Info :

Nutrition per Serving:
Calories: 130
Protein: 1g
Carbs: 32g
Fiber: 3g
Servings: 1
Cooking Time: 5 minutes

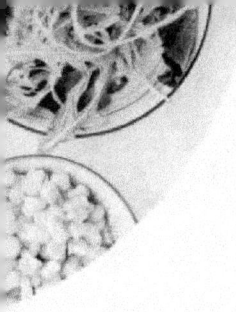

PUMPKIN PIE SMOOTHIE

INGREDIENTS

- 1/2 cup canned pumpkin (unsweetened)
- 1/2 cup almond milk (unsweetened)
- 1/2 tsp cinnamon
- 1 tbsp maple syrup

DIRECTIONS

1. Blend pumpkin, almond milk, cinnamon, and maple syrup until smooth.
2. Pour into a glass and serve chilled.
3. Enjoy a delicious, autumn-inspired dessert.

More Info :

Nutrition per Serving:
Calories: 110
Protein: 2g
Carbs: 20g
Fiber: 4g
Servings: 1
Cooking Time: 5 minutes

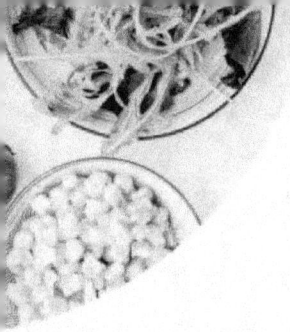

LEMON COCONUT ENERGY BITES

INGREDIENTS

- 1 cup shredded coconut (unsweetened)
- 2 tbsp lemon juice
- 1 tbsp maple syrup
- 1 tbsp chia seeds

DIRECTIONS

1. In a bowl, mix coconut, lemon juice, maple syrup, and chia seeds.
2. Form the mixture into small balls.
3. Refrigerate for 30 minutes to set.
4. Serve chilled as a zesty, energy-boosting snack.
5. Enjoy these refreshing bites.

More Info :

Nutrition per Serving:
Calories: 160
Protein: 3g
Carbs: 15g
Fiber: 4g
Servings: 2
Cooking Time: 5 minutes (plus chilling)

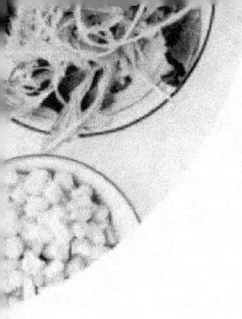

FROZEN BANANA POPS

INGREDIENTS

- 2 bananas (halved)
- 1/4 cup dark chocolate (dairy-free, melted)
- 2 tbsp shredded coconut (unsweetened)

DIRECTIONS

1. Insert popsicle sticks into banana halves.
2. Dip each banana in melted dark chocolate.
3. Sprinkle with shredded coconut.
4. Place on a tray and freeze for 2 hours.
5. Serve frozen for a healthy dessert.

More Info :

Nutrition per Serving:
Calories: 180
Protein: 2g
Carbs: 32g
Fiber: 5g
Servings: 2
Cooking Time: 5 minutes (plus freezing)

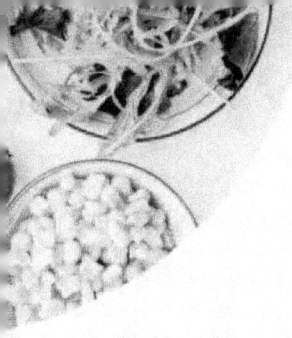

CHILLED BERRY
COMPOTE

INGREDIENTS

- 1/2 cup strawberries (sliced)
- 1/2 cup blueberries
- 1 tbsp maple syrup
- 1 tbsp lemon juice

DIRECTIONS

1. In a small saucepan, heat strawberries, blueberries, maple syrup, and lemon juice.
2. Simmer for 5 minutes until berries soften.
3. Let cool and chill in the fridge.
4. Serve as a topping for yogurt or on its own.

More Info :

Nutrition per Serving:
Calories: 80
Protein: 1g
Carbs: 20g
Fiber: 4g
Servings: 2
Cooking Time: 10 minutes (plus chilling)

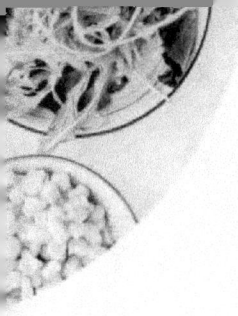

MAPLE ALMOND FUDGE

INGREDIENTS

- 1/4 cup almond butter
- 2 tbsp maple syrup
- 2 tbsp coconut oil (melted)
- 1/2 tsp vanilla extract

DIRECTIONS

1. Mix almond butter, maple syrup, melted coconut oil, and vanilla in a bowl.
2. Pour the mixture into a small lined dish.
3. Refrigerate for 2 hours until firm.
4. Slice into squares and serve.
5. Enjoy this creamy, no-bake fudge.

More Info :

Nutrition per Serving:
Calories: 160
Protein: 3g
Carbs: 10g
Fiber: 2g
Servings: 2-3
Cooking Time: 5 minutes (plus chilling)

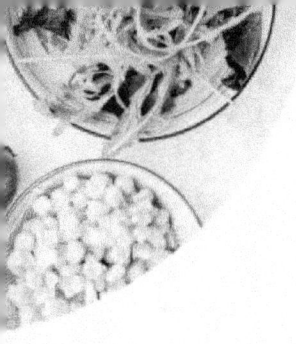

BAKED CINNAMON APPLES

INGREDIENTS

- 2 apples (cored and sliced)
- 1 tbsp maple syrup
- 1/2 tsp cinnamon
- 1 tbsp coconut oil (melted)

DIRECTIONS

1. Preheat oven to 350°F (175°C).
2. Toss apple slices with maple syrup, cinnamon, and melted coconut oil.
3. Place in a baking dish and bake for 20 minutes.
4. Serve warm as a comforting dessert.

More Info :

Nutrition per Serving:
Calories: 150
Protein: 0g
Carbs: 32g
Fiber: 6g
Servings: 1-2
Cooking Time: 25 minutes

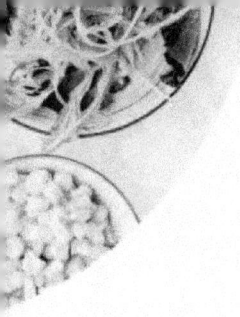

CHOCOLATE CHIA SEED PUDDING

INGREDIENTS

- 1/4 cup chia seeds
- 1 cup almond milk (unsweetened)
- 2 tbsp cocoa powder (unsweetened)
- 1 tbsp maple syrup

DIRECTIONS

1. Mix chia seeds, almond milk, cocoa powder, and maple syrup in a bowl.
2. Stir well and refrigerate for 4 hours or overnight.
3. Stir again before serving.
4. Enjoy a rich, chocolatey dessert.

More Info :

Nutrition per Serving:
Calories: 180
Protein: 5g
Carbs: 20g
Fiber: 10g
Servings: 2
Cooking Time: 5 minutes (plus chilling)

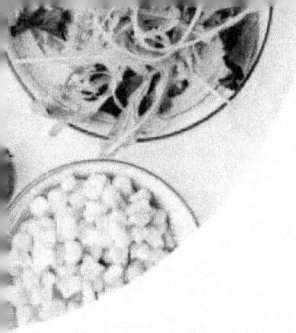

PEANUT BUTTER BANANA SMOOTHIE

INGREDIENTS

- 1 banana (frozen)
- 2 tbsp peanut butter (unsweetened)
- 1/2 cup almond milk (unsweetened)
- 1/2 tsp vanilla extract

DIRECTIONS

1. Blend banana, peanut butter, almond milk, and vanilla until smooth.
2. Pour into a glass and serve immediately.
3. Enjoy this creamy, protein-packed smoothie.

More Info :

Nutrition per Serving:
Calories: 210
Protein: 6g
Carbs: 30g
Fiber: 5g
Servings: 1
Cooking Time: 5 minutes

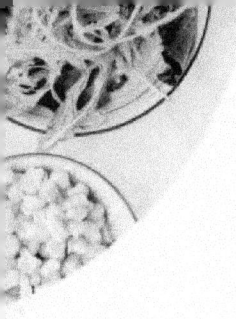

PUMPKIN COCONUT MUFFINS

INGREDIENTS

- 1/2 cup canned pumpkin (unsweetened)
- 1/2 cup gluten-free flour
- 1/4 cup shredded coconut (unsweetened)
- 1 tbsp maple syrup

DIRECTIONS

1. Preheat oven to 350°F (175°C).
2. Mix pumpkin, flour, coconut, and maple syrup in a bowl.
3. Spoon batter into a lined muffin tin.
4. Bake for 20 minutes until golden brown.
5. Let cool before serving.

More Info :

Nutrition per Serving:
Calories: 160
Protein: 3g
Carbs: 25g
Fiber: 4g
Servings: 3
Cooking Time: 25 minutes

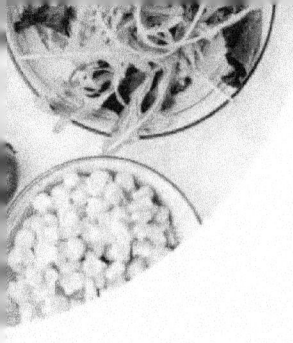

CINNAMON ALMOND GRANOLA

INGREDIENTS

- 1 cup gluten-free oats
- 1/4 cup slivered almonds
- 1 tbsp maple syrup
- 1/2 tsp cinnamon

DIRECTIONS

1. Preheat oven to 325°F (160°C).
2. Mix oats, almonds, maple syrup, and cinnamon in a bowl.
3. Spread on a baking sheet and bake for 15 minutes.
4. Let cool before serving as a crunchy dessert topping.

More Info :

Nutrition per Serving:
Calories: 180
Protein: 5g
Carbs: 25g
Fiber: 4g
Servings: 2
Cooking Time: 15 minutes

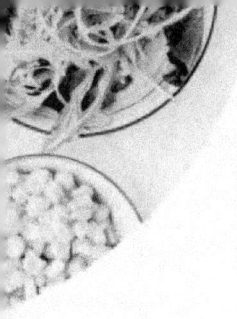

FROZEN GRAPES

INGREDIENTS

- 1 cup seedless grapes
- 1 tbsp lemon juice

DIRECTIONS

1. Rinse and dry the grapes.
2. Toss grapes with lemon juice.
3. Place on a baking sheet and freeze for 2 hours.
4. Serve frozen as a refreshing and naturally sweet dessert.

More Info :

Nutrition per Serving:
Calories: 70
Protein: 1g
Carbs: 18g
Fiber: 2g
Servings: 1
Cooking Time: 5 minutes (plus freezing)

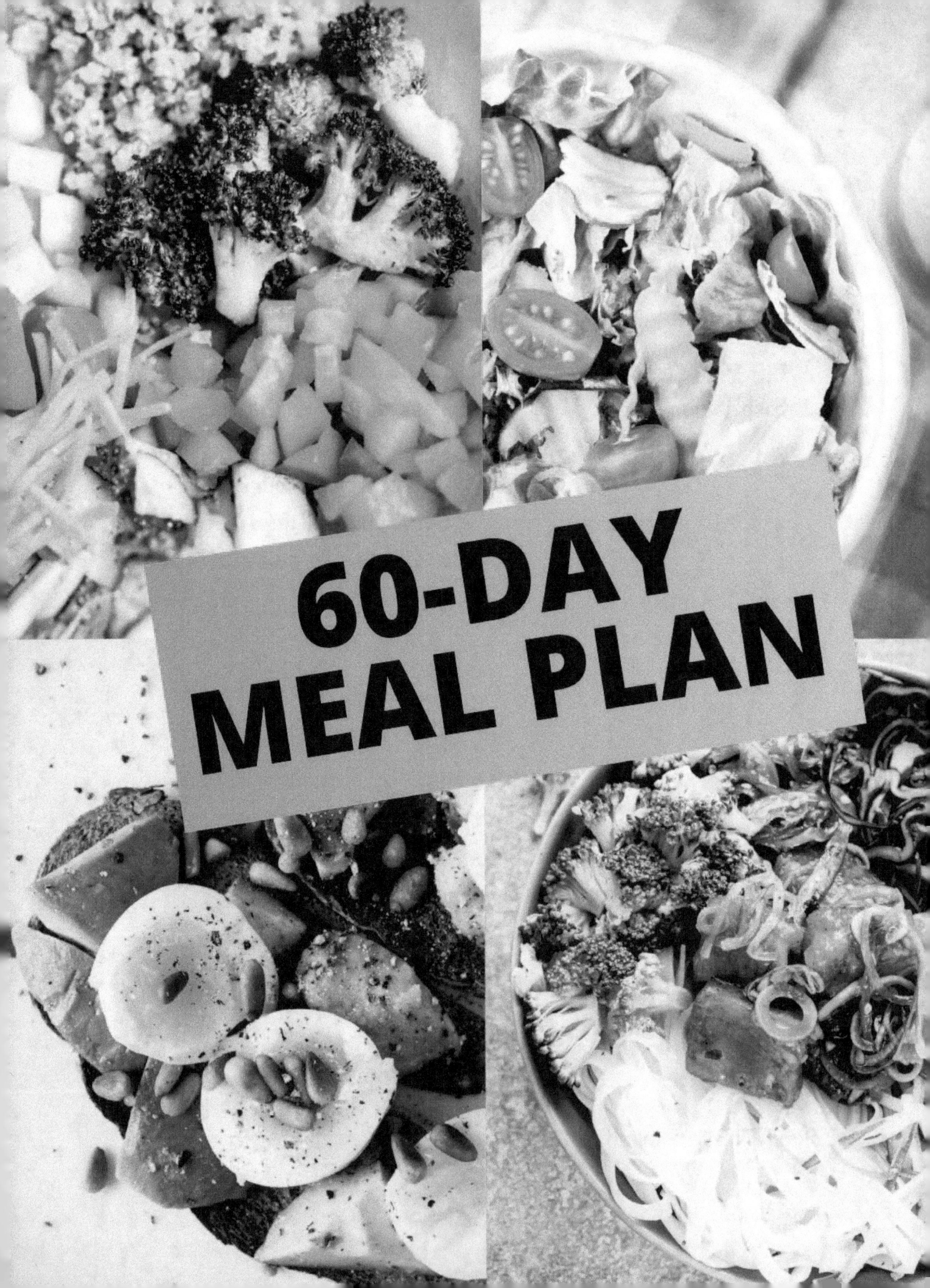

60-DAY MEAL PLAN

DAY 1

Breakfast: Banana Oat Pancakes
Lunch: Grilled Vegetable Quinoa Salad
Dinner: Vegetable Lentil Curry

DAY 2

Breakfast: Tofu Scramble
Lunch: Zucchini Noodles with Pesto
Dinner: Eggplant Stir-Fry

DAY 3

Breakfast: Chia Pudding
Lunch: Tofu Stir-Fry with Bok Choy
Dinner: Sweet Potato and Lentil Soup

DA 4

Breakfast: Quinoa Porridge
Lunch: Grilled Eggplant with Chickpeas
Dinner: Baked Tofu and Vegetable Skewers

DAY 5

Breakfast: Smoothie Bowl
Lunch: Avocado Chickpea Wrap
Dinner: Stuffed Bell Peppers with Quinoa

DAY 6

Breakfast: Zucchini Fritters
Lunch: Spinach and Feta Stuffed Portobello Mushrooms
Dinner: Chickpea and Spinach Stew

DAY 7

Breakfast: Coconut Yogurt with Berries
Lunch: Vegetarian Taco Salad
Dinner: Mushroom and Spinach Stir-Fry

DAY 8

Breakfast: Pumpkin Oatmeal
Lunch: Stuffed Zucchini Boats
Dinner: Zucchini and Mushroom Risotto

DA 9

Breakfast: Avocado Toast
Lunch: Rice Noodle Stir-Fry
Dinner: Roasted Sweet Potato and Quinoa Bowl

DAY 10

Breakfast: Buckwheat Pancakes
Lunch: Tomato and Avocado Wrap
Dinner: Lentil and Spinach Pasta

DAY 11

Breakfast: Polenta Porridge
Lunch: Cucumber Avocado Salad
Dinner: Vegetable and Tofu Skillet

DAY 12

Breakfast: Sweet Potato Breakfast Hash
Lunch: Roasted Vegetable Tacos
Dinner: Roasted Carrot and Lentil Salad

DAY 13

Breakfast: Eggplant Breakfast Wrap
Lunch: Lentil and Spinach Soup
Dinner: Baked Eggplant Parmesan

DA 14

Breakfast: Peanut Butter Chia Toast
Lunch: Quinoa and Roasted Veggie Bowl
Dinner: Grilled Zucchini and Chickpea Salad

DAY 15

Breakfast: Berry Coconut Smoothie
Lunch: Vegetarian Stuffed Bell Peppers
Dinner: Tofu and Vegetable Kebabs

DAY 16

Breakfast: Buckwheat Porridge
Lunch: Sweet Potato and Chickpea Salad
Dinner: Vegetable and Chickpea Stir-Fry

DAY 17

Breakfast: Overnight Oats
Lunch: Grilled Tofu with Veggies
Dinner: Roasted Veggie Tacos

DAY 18

Breakfast: Gluten-Free Waffles
Lunch: Eggplant and Lentil Stew
Dinner: Baked Sweet Potato Fries

DA 19

Breakfast: Coconut Rice Porridge
Lunch: Coconut Curry Vegetables
Dinner: Sweet Potato and Lentil Soup

DAY 20

Breakfast: Low-FODMAP Granola
Lunch: Vegetable Stir-Fry with Rice
Dinner: Roasted Sweet Potato and Quinoa Bowl

DAY 21

Breakfast: Smoothie Bowl
Lunch: Avocado Chickpea Wrap
Dinner: Zucchini and Mushroom Risotto

DAY 22

Breakfast: Pumpkin Oatmeal
Lunch: Cucumber Avocado Salad
Dinner: Vegetable Lentil Curry

DAY 23

Breakfast: Quinoa Porridge
Lunch: Grilled Eggplant with Chickpeas
Dinner: Tofu and Vegetable Kebabs

DA 24

Breakfast: Banana Oat Pancakes
Lunch: Vegetarian Taco Salad
Dinner: Baked Eggplant Parmesan

DAY 25

Breakfast: Zucchini Fritters
Lunch: Stuffed Zucchini Boats
Dinner: Chickpea and Spinach Stew

DAY 26

Breakfast: Tofu Scramble
Lunch: Spinach and Feta Stuffed Portobello Mushrooms
Dinner: Grilled Zucchini and Chickpea Salad

DAY 27

Breakfast: Chia Pudding
Lunch: Roasted Vegetable Tacos
Dinner: Mushroom and Spinach Stir-Fry

DAY 28

Breakfast: Coconut Yogurt with Berries
Lunch: Lentil and Spinach Soup
Dinner: Vegetable and Tofu Skillet

DA 29

Breakfast: Avocado Toast
Lunch: Zucchini Noodles with Pesto
Dinner: Sweet Potato and Lentil Soup

DAY 30

Breakfast: Buckwheat Pancakes
Lunch: Tofu Stir-Fry with Bok Choy
Dinner: Roasted Carrot and Lentil Salad

DAY 31

Breakfast: Coconut Rice Porridge
Lunch: Quinoa and Roasted Veggie Bowl
Dinner: Stuffed Bell Peppers with Quinoa

DAY 32

Breakfast: Sweet Potato Breakfast Hash
Lunch: Grilled Tofu with Veggies
Dinner: Baked Tofu and Vegetable Skewers

DAY 33

Breakfast: Eggplant Breakfast Wrap
Lunch: Cucumber Avocado Salad
Dinner: Vegetable Lentil Curry

DA 34

Breakfast: Peanut Butter Chia Toast
Lunch: Avocado Chickpea Wrap
Dinner: Roasted Veggie Tacos

DAY 35

Breakfast: Berry Coconut Smoothie
Lunch: Lentil and Spinach Soup
Dinner: Zucchini and Mushroom Risotto

DAY 36

Breakfast: Polenta Porridge

Lunch: Vegetarian Taco Salad

Dinner: Sweet Potato and Lentil Soup

DAY 37

Breakfast: Overnight Oats

Lunch: Tomato and Avocado Wrap

Dinner: Tofu and Vegetable Kebabs

DAY 38

Breakfast: Gluten-Free Waffles

Lunch: Spinach and Feta Stuffed Portobello Mushrooms

Dinner: Vegetable and Tofu Skillet

DA 39

Breakfast: Chia Pudding

Lunch: Grilled Vegetable Quinoa Salad

Dinner: Baked Eggplant Parmesan

DAY 40

Breakfast: Zucchini Fritters

Lunch: Stuffed Zucchini Boats

Dinner: Chickpea and Spinach Stew

DAY 41

Breakfast: Banana Oat Pancakes
Lunch: Quinoa and Roasted Veggie Bowl
Dinner: Mushroom and Spinach Stir-Fry

DAY 42

Breakfast: Tofu Scramble
Lunch: Cucumber Avocado Salad
Dinner: Grilled Zucchini and Chickpea Salad

DAY 43

Breakfast: Pumpkin Oatmeal
Lunch: Roasted Vegetable Tacos
Dinner: Vegetable Lentil Curry

DA 44

Breakfast: Smoothie Bowl
Lunch: Tomato and Avocado Wrap
Dinner: Baked Tofu and Vegetable Skewers

DAY 45

Breakfast: Coconut Yogurt with Berries
Lunch: Tofu Stir-Fry with Bok Choy
Dinner: Stuffed Bell Peppers with Quinoa

DAY 46

Breakfast: Quinoa Porridge
Lunch: Vegetarian Stuffed Bell Peppers
Dinner: Vegetable and Chickpea Stir-Fry

DAY 47

Breakfast: Avocado Toast
Lunch: Rice Noodle Stir-Fry
Dinner: Sweet Potato and Lentil Soup

DAY 48

Breakfast: Buckwheat Pancakes
Lunch: Lentil and Spinach Soup
Dinner: Zucchini and Mushroom Risotto

DA 49

Breakfast: Polenta Porridge
Lunch: Spinach and Feta Stuffed Portobello Mushrooms
Dinner: Roasted Carrot and Lentil Salad

DAY 50

Breakfast: Peanut Butter Chia Toast
Lunch: Avocado Chickpea Wrap
Dinner: Tofu and Vegetable Kebabs

DAY 51

Breakfast: Berry Coconut Smoothie
Lunch: Cucumber Avocado Salad
Dinner: Baked Eggplant Parmesan

DAY 52

Breakfast: Coconut Rice Porridge
Lunch: Grilled Tofu with Veggies
Dinner: Roasted Veggie Tacos

DAY 53

Breakfast: Chia Pudding
Lunch: Stuffed Zucchini Boats
Dinner: Mushroom and Spinach Stir-Fry

DA 54

Breakfast: Zucchini Fritters
Lunch: Tomato and Avocado Wrap
Dinner: Chickpea and Spinach Stew

DAY 55

Breakfast: Sweet Potato Breakfast Hash
Lunch: Zucchini Noodles with Pesto
Dinner: Vegetable and Tofu Skillet

DAY 56

Breakfast: Buckwheat Porridge
Lunch: Rice Noodle Stir-Fry
Dinner: Vegetable Lentil Curry

DAY 57

Breakfast: Banana Oat Pancakes
Lunch: Avocado Chickpea Wrap
Dinner: Grilled Zucchini and Chickpea Salad

DAY 58

Breakfast: Pumpkin Oatmeal
Lunch: Grilled Vegetable Quinoa Salad
Dinner: Roasted Sweet Potato and Quinoa Bowl

DA 59

Breakfast: Tofu Scramble
Lunch: Lentil and Spinach Soup
Dinner: Tofu and Vegetable Kebabs

DAY 60

Breakfast: Smoothie Bowl
Lunch: Coconut Curry Vegetables
Dinner: Zucchini and Mushroom Risotto

GROCERY LIST

GRAINS & STARCHES

- Oats (Banana Oat Pancakes, Pumpkin Oatmeal, Overnight Oats, Low-FODMAP Granola, Buckwheat Porridge)
- Buckwheat flour (Buckwheat Pancakes, Buckwheat Porridge)
- Quinoa (Quinoa Porridge, Grilled Vegetable Quinoa Salad, Quinoa and Roasted Veggie Bowl, Stuffed Bell Peppers with Quinoa)
- Rice (Coconut Rice Porridge, Vegetable Stir-Fry with Rice, Rice Noodle Stir-Fry)
- Polenta (Polenta Porridge)
- Rice noodles (Rice Noodle Stir-Fry)
- Gluten-free waffle mix (Gluten-Free Waffles)

DAIRY ALTERNATIVES

- Coconut yogurt (Coconut Yogurt with Berries)
- Lactose-free yogurt (Lactose-Free Yogurt Parfait)
- Almond milk (Various smoothies, Quinoa Porridge, Coconut Rice Porridge)

FRUITS

- Bananas (Banana Oat Pancakes, Chia Pudding, Peanut Butter Banana Smoothie, Banana Nice Cream, Frozen Banana Pops)
- Berries (Coconut Yogurt with Berries, Chia Pudding, Berry Coconut Smoothie, Frozen Berry Compote)
- Avocados (Avocado Toast, Cucumber Avocado Salad, Tomato and Avocado Wrap)
- Pumpkin (Pumpkin Oatmeal, Pumpkin Coconut Muffins, Pumpkin Pie Smoothie)
- Lemons (Lemon Coconut Energy Bites)
- Apples (Baked Cinnamon Apples, Apple Slices with Sunflower Seed Butter)
- Mango (Mango Sorbet)

NUTS & SEEDS

- Chia seeds (Chia Pudding, Coconut Chia Pudding, Chocolate Chia Seed Pudding)
- Almonds (Blueberry Almond Parfait)
- Coconut (Coconut Yogurt with Berries, Coconut Rice Porridge, Coconut Macaroons)
- Sesame seeds (Sesame Seed Crackers)

VEGETABLES

- Zucchini (Zucchini Fritters, Zucchini Noodles with Pesto, Stuffed Zucchini Boats, Zucchini and Mushroom Risotto)
- Sweet potatoes (Sweet Potato Breakfast Hash, Sweet Potato and Chickpea Salad, Sweet Potato and Lentil Soup, Baked Sweet Potato Fries)
- Eggplant (Eggplant Breakfast Wrap, Grilled Eggplant with Chickpeas, Eggplant Stir-Fry, Baked Eggplant Parmesan)
- Bell peppers (Vegetarian Stuffed Bell Peppers, Stuffed Bell Peppers with Quinoa)
- Cucumbers (Cucumber Avocado Salad, Cucumber Roll-Ups with Cream Cheese)
- Carrots (Roasted Carrot and Lentil Salad, Carrot Sticks with Peanut Butter)
- Spinach (Lentil and Spinach Soup, Chickpea and Spinach Stew, Spinach and Feta Stuffed Portobello Mushrooms)
- Portobello mushrooms (Spinach and Feta Stuffed Portobello Mushrooms)
- Bok choy (Tofu Stir-Fry with Bok Choy)
- Chickpeas (Avocado Chickpea Wrap, Roasted Chickpeas, Chickpea and Spinach Stew)

PROTEINS

- Tofu (Tofu Scramble, Tofu Stir-Fry with Bok Choy, Grilled Tofu with Veggies, Baked Tofu and Vegetable Skewers)
- Lentils (Lentil and Spinach Soup, Vegetable Lentil Curry, Sweet Potato and Lentil Soup)
- Peanut butter (Peanut Butter Chia Toast, Carrot Sticks with Peanut Butter, Peanut Butter Chocolate Bites)
- Sunflower seed butter (Apple Slices with Sunflower Seed Butter)
- Almond butter (Rice Cakes with Almond Butter)
- Chickpeas (Grilled Eggplant with Chickpeas, Chickpea and Spinach Stew, Roasted Chickpeas)

OILS & CONDIMENTS

- Olive oil (Grilled Vegetable Quinoa Salad, Various stir-fries)
- Coconut oil (Coconut Macaroons, Coconut Rice Porridge)
- Maple syrup (Maple Almond Fudge, Pumpkin Oatmeal)

HERBS, SPICES, & FLAVORINGS

- Cinnamon (Baked Cinnamon Apples, Cinnamon Almond Granola)
- Vanilla extract (Smoothie Bowls, Chia Pudding)
- Basil (Zucchini Noodles with Pesto)
- Curry powder (Coconut Curry Vegetables)
- Salt & Pepper (Various recipes)

SWEETENERS

- Honey (Smoothie Bowls, Chia Pudding)
- Maple syrup (Maple Almond Fudge, Overnight Oats)

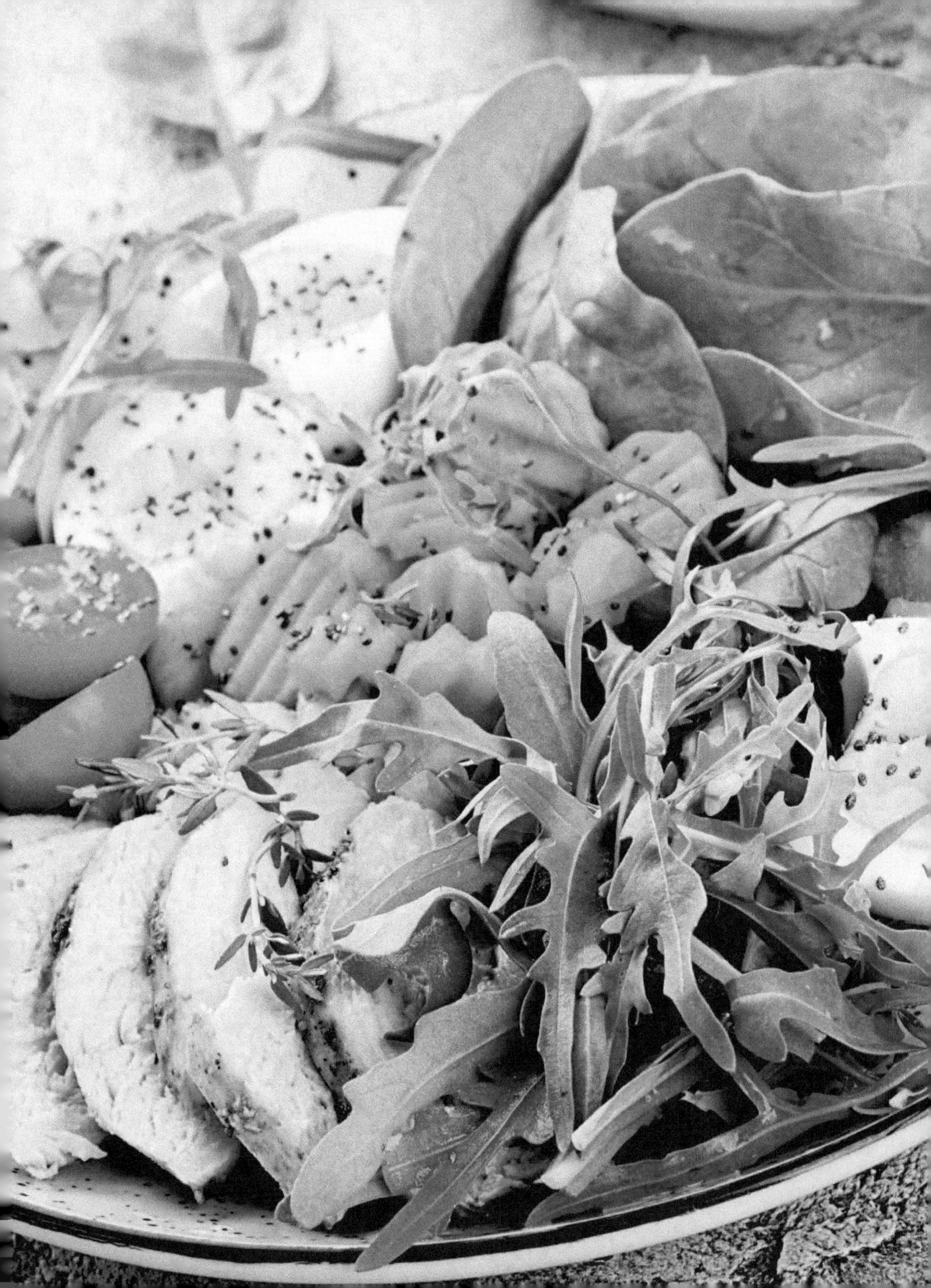

Conclusion

The Low FODMAP diet offers an effective and scientifically-backed approach to managing IBS and other digestive disorders, especially for vegetarians. While it may initially seem daunting due to the need to avoid many common plant-based foods, with thoughtful planning and substitutions, this diet can be both satisfying and nutrient-rich.

From delicious quinoa salads to nutrient-packed energy bites, the Low FODMAP vegetarian diet allows you to enjoy wholesome meals without triggering uncomfortable symptoms.

By focusing on low-FODMAP foods, you'll not only alleviate bloating, gas, and digestive discomfort but also enhance your overall well-being. As you embark on this journey, remember that relief is within reach. With patience and dedication, you can transform your digestive health and enjoy a variety of delicious meals.

Adopt the Low FODMAP vegetarian diet today, and take the first step towards reclaiming comfort and control over your body. You've got this!

WEEKLY MEAL

Planner

DATE

	BREAKFAST	LUNCH	DINNER	SNACKS
MONDAY				
TUESDAY				
WEDNESDAY				
THURSDAY				
FRIDAY				
SATURDAY				
SUNDAY				

WEEKLY MEAL

Planner

DATE

	BREAKFAST	LUNCH	DINNER	SNACKS
MONDAY				
TUESDAY				
WEDNESDAY				
THURSDAY				
FRIDAY				
SATURDAY				
SUNDAY				

WEEKLY MEAL
Planner

DATE

	BREAKFAST	LUNCH	DINNER	SNACKS
MONDAY				
TUESDAY				
WEDNESDAY				
THURSDAY				
FRIDAY				
SATURDAY				
SUNDAY				

WEEKLY MEAL

Planner

DATE

	BREAKFAST	LUNCH	DINNER	SNACKS
MONDAY				
TUESDAY				
WEDNESDAY				
THURSDAY				
FRIDAY				
SATURDAY				
SUNDAY				

WEEKLY MEAL
Planner

DATE

	BREAKFAST	LUNCH	DINNER	SNACKS
MONDAY				
TUESDAY				
WEDNESDAY				
THURSDAY				
FRIDAY				
SATURDAY				
SUNDAY				

WEEKLY MEAL

Planner

DATE

	BREAKFAST	LUNCH	DINNER	SNACKS
MONDAY				
TUESDAY				
WEDNESDAY				
THURSDAY				
FRIDAY				
SATURDAY				
SUNDAY				

WEEKLY MEAL
Planner

DATE

	BREAKFAST	LUNCH	DINNER	SNACKS
MONDAY				
TUESDAY				
WEDNESDAY				
THURSDAY				
FRIDAY				
SATURDAY				
SUNDAY				

WEEKLY MEAL
Planner

DATE

	BREAKFAST	LUNCH	DINNER	SNACKS
MONDAY				
TUESDAY				
WEDNESDAY				
THURSDAY				
FRIDAY				
SATURDAY				
SUNDAY				

WEEKLY MEAL

Planner

DATE

	BREAKFAST	LUNCH	DINNER	SNACKS
MONDAY				
TUESDAY				
WEDNESDAY				
THURSDAY				
FRIDAY				
SATURDAY				
SUNDAY				

WEEKLY MEAL

Planner

DATE

	BREAKFAST	LUNCH	DINNER	SNACKS
MONDAY				
TUESDAY				
WEDNESDAY				
THURSDAY				
FRIDAY				
SATURDAY				
SUNDAY				

THANK YOU
FOR READING!

THANK YOU FOR PURCHASING THE LOW FODMAP DIET FOR VEGETARIAN

I HOPE YOU FIND THE RECIPES BOTH ENJOYABLE AND HELPFUL ON YOUR CULINARY JOURNEY. YOUR FEEDBACK MEANS A LOT TO ME—PLEASE CONSIDER LEAVING AN HONEST REVIEW TO HELP OTHERS DISCOVER THE BOOK.

WARM REGARDS,

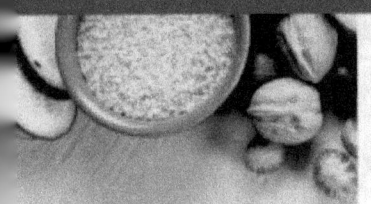
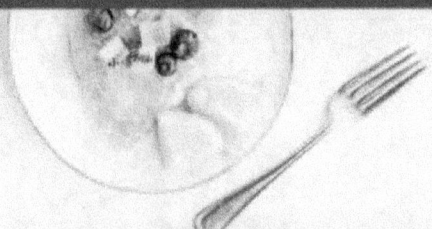
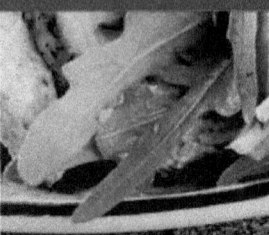

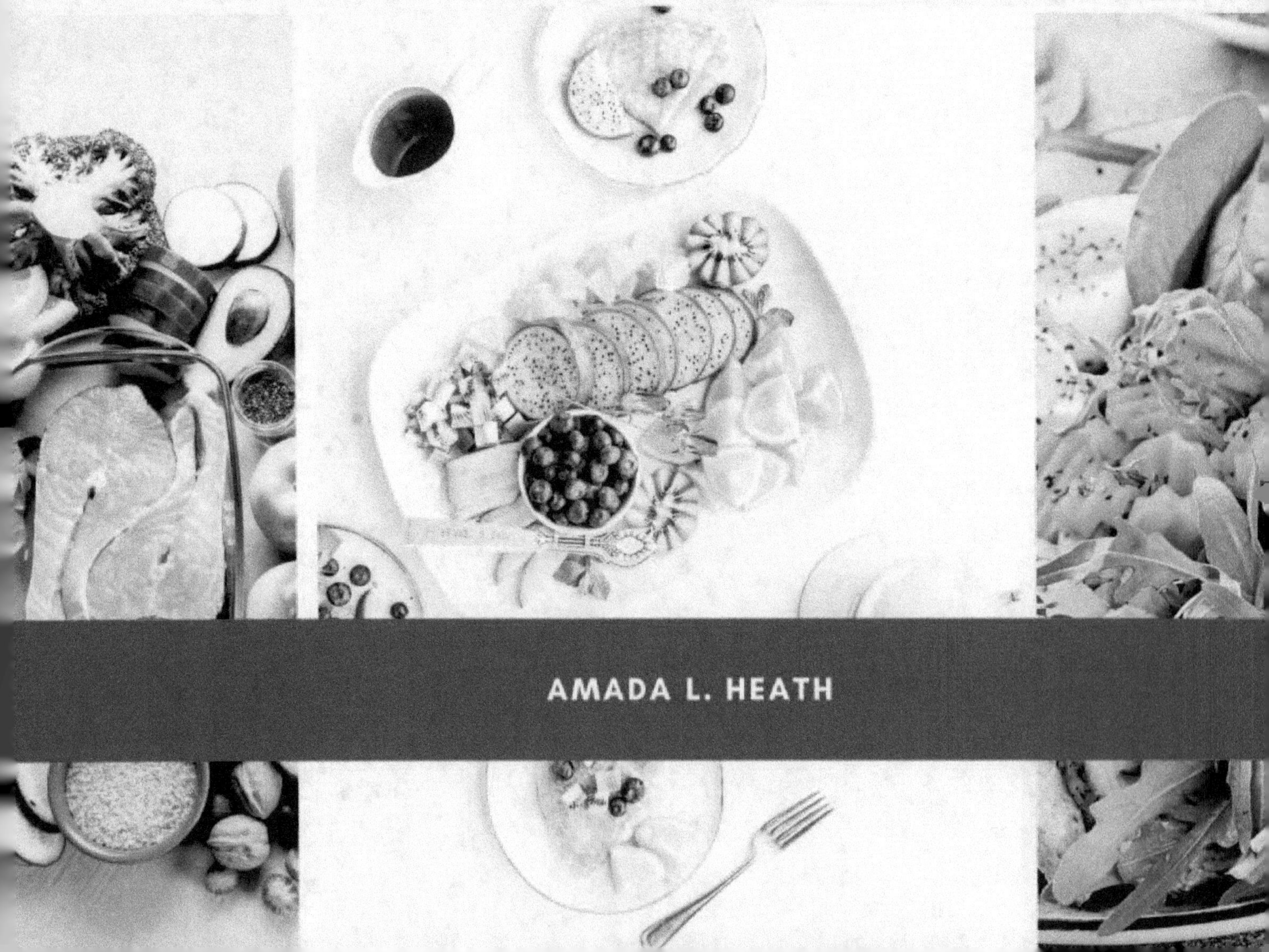

AMADA L. HEATH